BOHUNK'S REDEMPTION

From Blacking Out to Showing Up:
A Doctor's Adventures

By Bohunk

ISBN-13: 978-1-7338560-1-0
ISBN-13: 978-1-7338560-0-3

www.bohunksblog.com

Cover design by Francisca Ribeiro

Edited by R.H. and Christine Murphy

This is a memoir. The events, locales, and conversations are portrayed to the best of my memory. While all the stories in this book are true, some names and identifying details have been changed to protect the privacy of the people involved.

This book is not intended to be a substitute for the medical advice of a licensed physician. The reader should consult with their doctor in any matters relating to their health.

To those I love

and those I don't.

CONTENTS

BOHUNK'S REDEMPTION

From Blacking Out to Showing Up:
A Doctor's Adventures

PROLOGUE:
POWERFUL DRIVE WITHOUT WILLPOWER

*"You don't get to choose how you're going to die.
Or when. You can only decide how you're going
to live. Now."* —Joan Baez

I have only modest will power, but malignant drive. I will show you *how it was, what happened,* and *what it is like now,* and hopefully will not lecture you too much. From the abyss to the peak, I will relive my journey of recovery from death to life in my personal life and professional career for you. While I was born with predetermined genes, I had to test the environment to become a person I did not want to be. I engaged in an adventure, not knowing the outcome, and not caring about the future. But all that changed when I found hope, abundance and prosperity. If you read *Bohunk's Redemption,* I might very well tell your story.

This testimonial is true, *so help me God.* I will prove to you my life is better alive, as yours or someone you know, before it is too late. Yet, I don't reveal my identity beyond *Bohunk* to preserve my anonymity for enough humility to stay alive. Remember all that is not true is fiction anyway. All fiction is based on what is known, and all nonfiction does not replicate reality perfectly. I am on a mission from God, believe or not, real or imagined. Join me on my journey to happy destinies. And Bohunk thinks, therefore he is.

PART I.
WHAT IS WAS LIKE

1

HOPELESSNESS

*"The worst is not, so long as we can say,
'This the worst.'"* —William Shakespeare

*"The fact is that most alcoholics, for reasons yet obscure, have lost
the power of choice in drink. Our so-called willpower becomes practically non-existent. We are unable, at certain times, to bring into our
consciousness with sufficient force the memory of the suffering and
humiliation of even a week or a month ago. We are without defence
against the first drink."* —Twelve Steps and Twelve Traditions, Alcoholics Anonymous World Services, Inc.

I want you to know about my hopelessness. I hope you
never reach it, or maybe I do, to help you. That night I
either woke up or just was awake. I was in my usual intoxication of narcotics and tranquilizers, I am sure. I took them
in bottles around the clock. I don't recall any great emotion
or forethought as I left my bed in the Townhouse in Towson,
Maryland. I just gathered all my bottles of pills and walked
down the stairs to the kitchen. I opened the drawer and
picked the biggest kitchen knife I could find. I must have
filled a glass of water before I entered the stairs to the
dark basement. It's not like I thought a lot about suicide or
anything like that, but I just did it. I swallowed bottles of
pills to kill myself this time, probably the remainder of bottles of Valium, Quaalude, Darvon drugs, and I don't know
what else I had in my insane collection of poisons. Valium

is a tranquilizer I took to numb myself and treat other drug withdrawals, Quaalude is a potent sedative to knock myself out and trip into space, and Darvon, a narcotic I took daily in bottles to satisfy my addictive appetites; my desires for oblivion and stupor. I remember picking up the knife, but it turned out I didn't need to use it after all. You see, I lapsed into coma pretty quickly before I could complete the last suicidal act. At the time I not only wanted to kill myself, but I wanted to do it violently. A signature of my last stand I suppose, and how I felt. As it turned out, my lack of planning resulted in another self-defeat and failure.

I am sure you realize I did not walk or drive myself to the hospital. My wife at the time, for reasons unknown, woke up and noticed my bedroom light was on without me. She noticed I left a crack open in the basement door, so she went downstairs to take a look. There she found me unconscious and unresponsive, with empty pill bottles strewn around me on the floor. She noticed the knife and it dawned on her I needed immediate medical attention. She called the emergency service who took me to a local hospital, who quickly and sensibly, realized they could not save me from the pharmacopeia I had just ingested. They probably were also not too excited about dealing with not just another drug addict, but also a physician. Just my educated and experienced guess.

They concluded that I needed Man's Best Hospital, and lucky or not for us it was down the street, not too far away. Somehow they transported me, barely alive, to the Johns Hopkins Hospital where I was a Resident Physician in Psychiatry. Obviously, I was not awake for the trip, and would not know I had only left home, not earth itself, for days. I was in a deep coma on the ventilator in the Intensive Care Unit (ICU). I had taken far above the lethal dose of pills that dangerously bottomed out my blood pressure, threatened to shut down my kidneys, stop my heartbeats, and liquefy my brain. Much to my dismay at the time, my body remained intact and resisted destruction. My suicidal act was just another failed attempt by me in life.

Suddenly, I was thrust into a brief moment of consciousness by an overwhelming stroke of deep pain. I didn't, nor did they realize, that the doctors had inserted an elephant sized catheter in my bladder by mistake, as I lay in the intensive care unit at the Johns Hopkins Hospital. I also was not aware that Man's Best Hospital had performed a life saving procedure to drain and exchange my blood of the lethal quantities of depressant drugs, that had only been tried a few times in the world. As you would expect, I wasn't aware of anything while I was essentially and electrically brain dead, except that God awful pain which brought me briefly to life. Basically, they poured charcoal into my veins for the drugs to stick to long enough to filter out of my body. So a catheter was important you see, to run tons of fluid to displace the drugs.

My wife, Jennifer, knew I was an alcoholic when I met her. She also knew I did not want to attend Alcoholics Anonymous. So she said, "Try me instead." I jumped at the chance to yet again escape a real opportunity to stop drinking. She was quite older than I, but we married anyway. My best friend in high school and college, an attorney, gave me a free divorce as a wedding gift. He knew me and my problems. A cynical, but generous gift nonetheless, one that I later used *after* she saved my life and I sobered up. My story is that I met her in a compromised, intoxicated state. Even though she was a good woman, I did want to have children, and she was too advanced in years biologically. There were other reasons that operate to this day, including *me*.

A big part of this story is that I was a Resident in Psychiatry at the time, turned patient involuntarily, so to speak. I was told later that my Bostonian Irish Catholic Psychiatry Department Chair scolded the ICU team for their lackadaisical care of what they thought was a dirt ball drug addict who intentionally did this to himself. He was a fiery teacher who regularly exalted his followers to get them to see it his way. You might say I was a victim of the usual stigma drug addicts provoke and moralistic doctors on top of it. A double whammy. You can understand that to them, I was the cause of my impending death and deserved to die. I had self-inflicted my drug dependency, the addicting drugs the doctors prescribed had nothing to do with it. Just bad character and low morals, and too much of a good time. So much of a good time with drugs that they were killing me, or I killed myself for the fun of it.

I finally woke up looking up at nurses and doctors, figuring out I had failed again. I was alive. *How could this have happened?* More misery, disappointment, lying, deceit, and each day pouring pills down with no hope in sight. More failure, I felt. You must understand I was the grandson of immigrants who wanted me to succeed, to achieve more than they, to lift myself above them. That's why they worked so hard, tried to do the right things, to elevate me! All I did was bury their dreams in intoxicants.

The nurse taking care of me said, "You are a fighter, not a lover." What I did not know would happen was, punishment for my wrongdoings. I would spend the next few days in the ICU while I withdrew from my pills. The doctors who saved my life from a drug overdose were clueless how to treat drug withdrawal, not something taught to them in medical school or residency. I felt like an electrocuted cat, except I didn't die mercifully to end my wired state. I later learned I could have had seizures, delirium, and cardiac arrest from withdrawal from Valium, Quaaludes, and Narcotics. Instead I just suffered enough to teach me a lesson again. No way to get drugs for myself in an ICU, even if I asked for them. Back then, doctors and hospitals didn't pass out drugs on demand and request like they do now. Besides, they thought a doctor addict should probably suffer, just not die in Man's Best Hospital. A mantra I myself had used as Resident Physician, "Nobody dies on my service."

You ask, how did I end up on pills? Well, it started with alcohol. Many years of hard, blackout drinking. Beer first, then scotch, gin, sometimes day and night. It started in college at the University of Michigan and continued into medical school and residencies. I toured the country residency by residency, always escaping just before the hammer fell and my drinking would be found out. Never wanted to admit to anyone I had a drinking problem. Certainly, I did not want help, or to stop drinking, despite worsening trouble.

As a medical student, I had a problem with premature ejaculation from alcohol withdrawal, and my favorite medical school professor prescribed Valium to calm me, to delay my ejaculation. While it worked initially, little did I know I would later use it for alcohol withdrawal daily, until I could get more alcohol. I would take 5 mg tablets, 4 to 8 or more at a time, several times throughout the day. Then I'd drink almost a fifth of liquor or 6 to 12 beers, often alcohol fortified malt liquor. As you might expect, I had trouble getting up in the morning, and often not on time. And in an awful state of mind and body, terrible anxiety and shakes, therefore the treatment was Valium, another addicting drug to substitute for alcohol. Valium is really, chemically, alcohol in a pill form.

Somehow, and I can't remember why, I started pre-scribing myself Darvon (propoxyphene), a scheduled nar-cotic (opioid) with Valium because it made me drowsy and foggy. I didn't want to keep asking doctors to prescribe so many pills. Besides, they probably would have said no years ago. Maybe not now. I had to stay awake sometimes 24-36 hours at a time when on call as a Resident in Medi-cine, and couldn't afford to fall asleep talking to patients or not wake up when the nurse called me for an emergency. Darvon cut the withdrawal symptoms, even energized me, and substituted that God awful addictive drive for alcohol or other drugs.

I thought often of using alcohol intravenously (inject-ing into my veins), because it was so hard to swallow ini-tially, due to its terrible taste in the morning and irritation. I never liked the taste of liquor, and besides the bloating, beer was only tolerable. I drank for intoxication, barely for euphoria in the beginning; later for oblivion and stupor without good feelings. Never much enjoyment from alcohol and drugs, mostly just hard work and pain. Both were like poison, and a shit sandwich, yet I struggled for another bite, risking my life, liberty, and pursuit of happiness, every day. And not much chance to quit, on my own.

As with alcohol and Valium 20 mg to 100 mg per day, I took bottles of 100 mg Darvon capsules a day, 50 to a 100 capsules handful at times, not really keeping count. This made me busy going from pharmacy to pharmacy, writing prescriptions for myself and wife. My wife was in a lot of pain as was I, so I had to have a lot of Darvon. I also may have lifted pills from the hospital while I was on duty, thoughtlessly depriving patients of their pain relief perhaps. I can still recall swallowing gobs of pills and drain-ing bottles of them.

My first sponsor in Alcoholics Anonymous, a physician himself, said he had never seen anyone, patient or addict, take so many pills at a time, and did not understand how I could still be alive. He said I was the sickest person he had ever seen in AA. I told him it was easy, just become addicted, prescribe to myself as a physician, and work long hours as a resident. I explained I could make it to class and the hospital intoxicated on pills, and it was a lot harder, if not impossible, to do that drinking as much alcohol as I did. After all, I didn't want to get caught, and could not predict how much I would drink but I knew I would drink, or what I would say or do intoxicated on alcohol. Although I knew I could think on drugs, it was still noticeable to others. Alcohol intoxication was too obvious, smelled, so I looked worse intoxicated on alcohol than drugs, if you can believe that.

I forgot to mention at the beginning of this morbid story, I was not new to suicide attempts, as I had tried on other occasions. Besides living a life of slowly progressive death in mind and body due to alcohol and drugs, I once tried to end my life more abruptly. While on a date with a nurse I had met in the hospital, I cut my wrists with a kitchen knife. I was never interested in surgery as a medical student or resident so I happened to miss the radial artery in my attempt. You should know the radial nerve runs close to the radial artery, and because I didn't attempt suicide under anesthesia other than alcohol, it hurt like hell when I hit the nerve. The pain stopped further dissection, and the bleeding probably obscured my surgical field, not to mention my alcohol intoxication.

Surprisingly, I never saw my suicide coming, I didn't plan it that night, I just up and did it. Like my use of alcohol, my suicide attempt was compulsive and unpredictable. I don't think my date and I even had a fight, not sure what provoked it other than alcohol and fatigue, as I'm sure I had been on call without sleep during my medical internship. Maybe I got upset because she declined my sexual advances, I don't remember, as usual.

I was rushed to the University of Michigan Hospital, where I woke up on the Orthopedic Floor with a broken mind, not fractured bones. My Chairman of Medicine, a wonderful man, wanted to spare me the embarrassment of being a spectacle on a medical floor where I worked as medical resident, and after all a cut wrist was surgical, and not medical. The next morning during rounds he said, "You have a disease, like a broken bone, and we will treat it as doctors." I wish I had heard him then, but I was not the least bit interested in admitting I had an addictive disease. How do you figure I would not agree with him, sitting in a bed in my hospital gown, where I am a resident, looking pretty sick with a bandage on my poorly self-inflicted injury?

Another spuriously proud part of my story is that I was arrested for drunk driving four times within six months after arriving in Ann Arbor to serve my internship. I rationalized I suffered from a lack of sleep, though I had a blood alcohol level of 0.22, almost three times the legal limit in Michigan. Here I was, at the zenith of my aspirations, a young medical resident in a prestigious program, waking up in the County jail. I assure you I didn't plan on facing the judge in the morning in my day old clothes after a night's sleep in jail; unshaven, shaking, and tremulous from alcohol withdrawal. Worse, I was supposed to be on rounds in the hospital, something an intern never missed no matter what, under no circumstances, ever! Patients were sick, and dying, and I was supposed to care for them as the frontline doctor. The intern in a medical residency is the linchpin, the doctor closest to the patient, most responsible and knowledgeable, and accountable. Not being there was a disgrace and a blow to my pride, let alone compromising patient care. The judge didn't really take pity on my insolence, but did release me to the catch up with my medical team in the afternoon. Just another blip from my helpless and humiliating alcoholism. I repeated this embarrassing debacle three more times. Not too smart for a medical intern.

Back to my coma. Months before my overdose, I had dropped from 200 to 140 lbs., with a severe loss of appetite. I regularly disimpacted my rectum with gloves due to narcotic anorexia and constipation. Not to mention how goofy I looked and sounded on these drugs. My mentors in Psychiatry Department at Hopkins were always asking questions, "Are you sure you are not taking drugs?" and, "Of course not," I responded. Another curious benefit from the narcotics was I did not have to drink alcohol nearly as much. I was able to substitute drugs for alcohol, so I could say I was not drinking. However, that would backfire, as I remember when I was administering electroconvulsive shock therapy for depression to a patient, I'd not be able to stand up, as I was under the influence of chloral hydrate, another potent sedative I sometimes took for reasons God only knows. I didn't like it too much because it caused my nose to itch and my eyes to water a noxious intoxication. And I had to respond to too many questions about my health, namely drug use. Surprisingly, no one actually drug tested me, though, I am sure they thought of it. Maybe they wouldn't know what to do if they found drugs. Our Psychiatry Chair was very loyal, and I'm sure he did not want to expose me or jeopardize my career or patient care.

Because you are reading this book, you know I survived and finally quit for good, drugs, and alcohol. But you don't know how I got here from there, and where there even started. Maybe Adam or Eve, or both had genes for alcoholism and drug addiction. They did show signs of compulsive behaviors, unable to resist apples and sin and all. My disease certainly looked and felt like sin, and made me do immoral things. Thus, I looked like I had a morality problem, as did Adam and Eve. I certainly did want to use drugs and alcohol, but did not want to die, or hurt so many others, or fail at so many things like showing up. I wanted to be a contender. Where did I go wrong, what made me drink so much, and use so many drugs, so often? Did I have deep rooted psychological problems? Was I a sinner, have bad character, raised wrong, beaten, deprived, poor, rude, ugly, psychopathic, mentally ill? The answer to all these questions is yes, and no.

Addiction to drugs and alcohol is observable by an incessant preoccupation with acquiring them, continued use despite adverse consequences, and a pattern of relapse. Or, boiled down, I kept seeking and using alcohol and drugs despite continued and repeated jackpots, jails, no shows, suicides, broken promises, and failed responsibilities. As I sought alcohol, and later drugs, I went to any length to get them. Expected and repeated bad consequences followed, essentially turning me into an "ass." Although I would swear off alcohol almost daily, I would pursue it and become intoxicated hours later. I can recall daily trips to the liquor store, saying to myself, *I will quit tomorrow.* Saying it over and over again, tomorrows after tomorrows. Talk about a preoccupation; I was rarely without alcohol. Why I didn't store more alcohol than a day's supply was because I really wanted to quit, and tried to do it daily, but was carried away and compelled by the insane drive to use. So I continued, regardless of the serious and dangerous consequences.

To this day, I am not sure why I became intoxicated,

as I had little conscious awareness during it, and spent much of my inebriated years unaware, in a blackout mental state. An alcoholic blackout is life not lived, no recording of the conscious experience, no memory trace created. A blackout is less than sleeping, as sleep is still a mental experience, whereas a blackout is no mental experience. They say, insanity is doing the same thing over and over again, expecting different results. I say, if blackout drinking is not insanity, then there is no such thing as insanity. But I didn't learn or could not connect early on, that intoxication led to many disappointments, lost opportunities, delays, harrowing near death experiences.

What is really the kicker, and whoever figures it out should win the Nobel Prize, is why I went back, why I relapsed so often. I could quit from time to time, but I could not stay quit. I always went back to the drug or drink despite having the same or worse problems, over and over and over again. I really believe I drank against my will, not because I enjoyed it, or found relief in it. I became so depressed and anxious, and had so much pain, because I used alcohol and drugs obsessively.

Before I start my journey into the present, I want to explain how powerfully addicting and dangerous the drugs are that I used. I will tell you, I did not take them as prescribed. But taking them as prescribed does not make the drugs less addicting. I also want you to have confidence in what I say about my drug use. Cynically, I am happy to report I achieved an almost perfect score on my Pharmacology Test as part of the National Board Examination for medical licensing. I scored 798 out of a possible 800 points or in the 99 percentile among all medical students at the time in the US. I guess you could say practical experience or applied knowledge helped, but I also had a really good teacher in medical school to match my mental and physical affinity for drugs. Since I prescribed them, I took them however I wanted to, or whenever my addiction to them demanded. But what they did to me, and others chemically, was to capture and control.

In fact, some of what I used are no longer legal to manufacture, while others remain on the market to addict millions of victims. In my case, I became almost psychotic, very aggressive when I took Quaaludes (methaqualone), and they certainly sedated me. Quaaludes are classified as depressants because they suppress the central nervous system or brain. I was mostly a "downer" kind of guy, preferring to be sedated than stimulated. Quaaludes would depress me into a foggy state with a complete mental disconnect from reality. I turned into a strange, out of this world character, separated from rational thinking and acting.

Originally intended for sleep, Quaaludes quickly gained popularity in the 1960s and 1970s as "ludes," and later as a date rape drug. Bill Cosby is alleged to have used it as a knockout for his various sexual offenses. The drug was withdrawn from the market and identified as a Schedule I drug from the Drug Enforcement Administration (DEA) in the U.S., meaning it has no legitimate medical purpose, and is highly addicting and dangerous. Among the effects of overdose are delirium, convulsions, hypertonia, hyperreflexia, vomiting, kidney failure, coma, and death through cardiac or respiratory arrest. A standard tablet adult dose of Quaaludes was 300 mg, but I think I took 500 mg tablets, and a lethal dose is 8000 mg or 16 pills, or as little as 2000 mg or 4 pills.

I remember taking a better part of a bottle of an unknown number of Quaalude pills in my suicidal overdose.

I usually filled prescriptions for large quantities of pills because I swallowed so many. You understand I ingested enough to probably kill me many times. The drug persists for days in the blood stream, making it a difficult drug to filter from your system in the ICU. But my psychoanalyst said to me, after I survived the overdose and cardiac intensive unit, "You are like a cat with nine lives." I can tell you, I used up quite a few lives, taking pills.

As I mentioned before, I substituted Darvon for drinks since I became too intoxicated from alcohol, losing complete control of thoughts and actions. I don't remember how many Darvon I took in my lethal overdose, but my custom was handfuls a day. I counted my self-prescribing in handfuls, not tablets or capsules. Darvon is the brand name for propoxyphene which was an analgesic in the opioid category. Opioid drugs are narcotics based on their chemical structure and clinical effects. Thus, why I spent time in the cardiac intensive unit for monitoring.

Darvon is called an opioid pain reliever and was potent when I took handfuls of 100 mg capsules per day. It was also used to treat withdrawal from other opioids such as heroin and morphine. An overdose from Darvon is no lovelier than ludes, causing central nervous depression, respiratory depression, seizures, decreased heart rate and contractility and electrical conductivity, and failure, aspiration pneumonia, and altering thoughts and mood. Darvon was eventually taken off the market due to fatal overdoses and heart arrhythmias (abnormal heart rhythms), but not in time for me. As you might expect I spent most of my days on a life and death high wire, bombed and blowing in the wind.

In 2009, the Federal Drug Agency (FDA), voted against the continued marketing of propoxyphene based on its weak pain killing abilities, addictiveness, association with fatal heart problems, and risks of overdose and deaths. Darvon carried a black box warning which was to emphasize a hazardous point about the medication, "Propoxyphene should be used with extreme caution, if at all, in patients who have a history of substance/drug/alcohol abuse, depression with suicidal tendency, or who already take medications that cause drowsiness (sedatives, tranquilizers)." Fatalities occurred in such patients when propoxyphene was misused.

In 2010, the FDA requested the cessation of all sale of Darvon from the U.S. market due to heart arrhythmia in patients who took the drug. I point out that they did not take the drug off the market due to its high addictiveness. As if addiction is not a major, lethal problem. My guess is that there would have been so many heart related deaths if addicted people did overuse Darvon, as I did. And Darvon in normal, nonaddicted doses was probably not a high risk cardiac drug. Propoxyphene was a Schedule I substance, highly addicting, and dangerous. As usual, the FDA and doctors don't get how lethal addiction is, and its role in large numbers of drug related deaths from many causes and overdose.

Valium is generic diazepam, and a benzodiazepine, which is not an innocuous tranquilizer. Little did I know that Valium's side effects include suicide, sedation, memory loss, lasting anxiety, depression, cognitive problems, and neurological symptoms. Valium increases propensity for self-harm, and as in my case of overdose, it added to the sedative effects of other medications which caused respiratory depression. Tolerance, dependence, and addiction regularly occur in repeated use. Withdrawal symptoms are common, 50-100% of users, and was so in me. I had severe anxiety, depression, and suicidal thinking for a year or two after I stopped using Valium. Even a year after I had stopped using it, I was looking for a big truck to just run me over. Overdose and intoxication made me drowsy, confused; with impaired coordination, walking, talking, and you guessed it, coma. It was especially lethal if taken with other drugs, opioids, and sedatives, as I did.

As most addicting drugs go, they are very popular with both physicians and patients. Year after year, hydrocodone and opioid medications like propoxyphene are the most commonly prescribed and sold medications of any medications in the U.S. Opioid drugs are in the top 20 drugs prescribed and sold. Benzodiazepines as well. Most addicting drugs dwarf others in number of prescribed medications. More than medications for blood pressure, diabetes, or antibiotics. You ask, why? Is it because pain is such a common problem? I doubt it, although pain is a common complaint. Opioids are not effective in the treatment of long lasting, chronic pain. They did little to solve pain for me, rather instead, *creating* pain of all kinds, physical and mental. And I know others. The answer is ADDICTION, and its powerfully lethal, compulsive hold on people. Addiction is like a cancer that overpowers and destroys its host.

Of course, pharmaceutical companies who gain billions of dollars of profit, not only attempt to fill the addictive appetite but also push these addicting medications in advertisements and with financial support of corrupt doctors. I once tried to find a medical conference not supported by a pharmaceutical company, without success. Drug companies are everywhere, and control the medical profession and hospitals. Even my doctors are still trying to put me on drugs that don't really help, and have offered me Vicodin despite my morbid history of drug addiction. They think *I'm* crazy because I don't want their poisons.

Remember what the dormouse said
Feed your head, feed your head

—"White Rabbit" Jefferson Airplane

2

WHY ME? A VICTIM? A PERPETRATOR?
(Family, Religion, Divorce)

"No one is content with his own lot."
—Horace

Y ou might say I was born into a death trap. Although I became an addict, I was still a victim. I did not cause my addiction or will it to happen. I blame my journey to the brink of death on my genes, and will tell you about them. And maybe environment helped determine my destiny, though not completely, if you believe in free will. You understand I came from a family history of alcoholism; drugs were not a big thing back then. My mother and three of her four brothers and sisters were alcoholics, three died of alcoholic complications. She herself died of strokes, from heart disease complicated by alcohol. My father died drinking alcohol, and spent his last years depressed in lonely drinking. He stopped taking his heart medications and died of a cardiac arrest, alcohol having robbed him of his will to live. When I asked that they not drink while with me and my daughters, they both chose the bottle over family. We did not visit him much as he drank himself to death in his later years. The power of alcohol was too much, though I know he loved us.

I think my paternal grandfather was a bootlegger in

New York City. He was certainly involved with alcohol. And I don't know much about my maternal grandfather who died at a young age of something mysterious. Neither of my grandmothers drank.

All of my grandparents were immigrants to the United States. All arrived legally through Ellis Island and passed the Statute of Liberty. I am the typical American mutt. Both my mother's parents were born in and immigrated from Lithuania before it fell under Russian control. Her father was a farmer, and her mother raised their five children. They came over in the large wave of Eastern Europeans, and given opportunities for settlement to farm in Michigan. My mother was often evasive about my heritage. When I asked her, she simply said, "You are an American." No matter how many ways I presented the questions, she would not talk about the nationality of her parents, although she knew. She thought I would do better in the U.S. as an American, and that being Lithuanian would only help in Lithuania. She felt strongly in integration to succeed. None of her relatives talked much about the "old country." We certainly didn't talk about alcoholism. Not something she believed in, even when I almost killed myself from it and drug addiction. She was kind hearted and understood other illnesses, but not addiction. She could control herself, except in her drinking. She was an alcoholic.

According to my mother, she left the farm at the age of 14. She said she disliked the farm life and didn't particularly get along with her old school mother, who could barely speak English through her heavy Lithuanian dialect. My mother said she lived by herself and worked in factories. And eventually put herself through school to learn "bookkeeping," and go on to work as a secretary. There is a large gap I don't know about from the time she was age 14 until she married at the age of 28. She talked little about her life actually. I do recall she lamented over the years that her mother prevented her from accepting a college scholarship offered her by a rich neighbor. She said she did very well as a student in her one room schoolhouse, and regretted the opportunity to graduate from college, to better herself. That is something she demanded of us, and left to my sister and I.

But I was never too proud of my farm heritage, which did not blend in well with my newfound ambition for high society. I was not proud of my Jewish heritage, but wanted to be part of a more esteemed Anglo Saxon, Protestant status, and in fact I was downright ashamed of my mother at times. She did not yet speak correct English, or carry herself with the level of class I aspired to. You could call me a snob, and I probably was and still am. Always feeling above the next guy, wanting to outdo them. Many of my friends' parents graduated from college or came from established, old American families. Whereas I came from "immigrants," whose offspring were still not educated or well spoken. Though many people complimented my mother for her outgoing personality and charm, at the time I only saw her basic flaws and shortcomings. She never graduated from high school, worked as secretary, and married a Jew. What more do I have to say? Alcohol may have been a way to raise my status, and blot out my inferior makings, from a plain family's broken English, and ploughed fields.

According to my mother, my father on the other hand, was a handsome, suave man from the big city. He was born in the Bronx, New York to Jewish immigrants. He was definitely more presentable to me, but he was Jewish and weighed over 300 lbs., at 6 feet and 1 ½ inches. His nickname was "Tiny." Back then, he was a big man, and still would be today, I suppose. He was a car salesman, and later owned automobile agencies. I wasn't too high on fast talking salesmen. In fact, I wasn't too high on business, which I thought was beneath me. I broke my father's heart the day he wanted me to join him in a car business he owned, and told him I wanted to stay in and graduate from college instead. I don't know if I felt that opportunity was beneath me or if I wanted to continue to drink and dream and wander, in philosophy and psychology classes instead. And maybe become a physician. I was determined to show I was better. All the wrong reasons to become a doctor, but it was the American way. To develop a superiority complex and succeed where predecessors did not! More about my ever-present competitiveness...

My father's Jewish mother was born and immigrated from Romania in the early nineteen hundreds and settled in the Bronx. His Jewish father was born in Poland and immigrated to New York City as well, and according to my grandmother, he was a "bum." Neither seemed particularly educated or accomplished in careers. My grandfather died at a young age, and distinguished himself as a cigar maker and probable bootlegger. Otherwise, I was not given much more information about him. My grandmother spoke in broken English her entire life, maintaining her strong Romanian accent. She worked as a seamstress in the sweatshops in New York, but didn't talk much about it. Nobody talked about their past. Just what was I going to become.

My grandparents carried on the tradition of my entire immigrant family by not extending or reciting with me their European history, but rather pushed me towards integration into American society. At that time there was not much government influence, support, or intrusion in their lives. They were pretty dependent on their own determination and resources, and were committed to integration as the best way to share the American values and opportunities, to get ahead. They were focused on my "bettering myself;" *work hard, be honest, become educated.* Heavy emphasis on doing it the right way. Not much else I can recall. I do remember a meeting with my grandmother saying to me during my struggling drinking days, "What's wrong with you, you are not finished with college, not married, do not have a job." She didn't mention my drinking. I cried in front of her because it was all true, and she said it in such a serious, judgmental manner, yet concerned. When she saw me crying, she asked in her Romanian accent, "I shouldn't care?" then laughed and invited me to lunch as she usually did. She is the same person who called my grandfather and father "bums." I don't know if alcoholism was a problem for my grandfather, but it was for my father. My Jewish Polish grandfather died early. You figure it out.

In a 2014 *USA Today* article, "The Heaviest-Drinking Countries In The World" it reveals the following:

Nearly all of the countries with the highest levels of alcohol consumption are located in Eastern Europe. They include Russia and other former Soviet Union nations such as Belarus, Lithuania, Moldova, and Ukraine. The only top-consuming nation not located in Eastern Europe is Andorra, a principality located between France and Spain in the Pyrenees. Five of the heaviest drinking countries also had among the 10 highest prevalence of alcoholism. These include alcoholism and other forms of health-damaging use of alcohol. Such disorders lead to physical problems such as liver cirrhosis and mental illnesses such as depression. The three nations with the highest rates of alcoholism, Hungary, Russia, and Belarus, were all among the 10 heaviest drinking nations

[...] In Romania, life expectancy at birth is 68.7 years [...] Drinking rates among younger Romanians were particularly high. More than 37% of teenagers between 15 and 19 years old had engaged in binge drinking in the last 30 days, more than in all but a handful of countries. As is usually the case, alcohol consumption was more of an issue among males — more than 55% of Romanian men ages 15 to 19 said they had engaged in binge drinking in the previous 30 days, considerably higher than most other countries. Binge drinking may be associated with alcohol related fatalities in the county. Nearly 9% of all deaths in 2012 were alcohol related, more than in all but a handful of nations.

In the aptly titled *Guardian* article, "Last Orders for Lithuanian Teenagers As Government Cracks Down on Alcohol," it states,

According to the latest World Health Organization data, Lithuanians are the world's heaviest drinkers and the country's addiction shows no signs of abating. In 2016, Lithuanians drank, on average, the equivalent of 18.2 litres of pure alcohol per person, up from 14.9 litres more than a decade ago. That is the same as 9-10 large beers (500ml) or medium glasses of wine (152ml) over the year, equating to two-and-a-half glasses a day.

Relevant to me, *The Baltic Times* article "Lithuania Still Suicide Capital" declares,

Lithuania once again takes the dubious honor of being the country with the highest suicide rate in the world, according to figures released this week - and the gap between it and the rest of the world is huge. The news from the Lithuanian Statistics Department is disheartening. Lithuanians commit suicide more often than anyone else in the world. While last year's numbers have decreased slightly from 2000, they remain an almost two-fold increase compared with 10 years ago. Lithuania leads the world, with 44 citizens out of every 100,000 taking their own lives. Russia is second with 39. Estonia and Latvia are third and fourth with 38 and 36. The average in the European Union is 20. "Around 80 percent of suicides are alcohol-related, and we see the biggest problems with that in the countryside. In rural areas, everybody drinks."

The aforementioned *USA Today* piece concludes,

Of the 3.3 million alcohol related deaths worldwide, a third were caused by cardiovascular diseases and diabetes. Unintentional injuries accounted for 17.1% of alcohol-related deaths. Various types of cancer, gastrointestinal diseases, and intentional self-harm were also common causes of deaths related to alcohol. In five of these nations, 30% of deaths in 2012 were alcohol related, compared to 5.9% of deaths worldwide. Life expectancies in the nations with heavy alcohol use are also shorter. The average life expectancy at birth in high income nations was 79.3 years as of 2012, far higher than in almost all of the heaviest drinking nations. In Romania, the average life expectancy was just 68.7 years. In Russia and Ukraine the average life expectancy was below 72 years as well.

My mother met my father in Miami, Florida, where she was working as a waitress at the time. She was an adventuresome soul, not beholden to the established life, certainly not the old country. He was on furlough from the United States Army during World War II, and just happened to be visiting the area. She said, "He was so handsome, tall, and polished with New York accent and mannerisms." She, who still had some country dialect, was instantly attracted to this ambitious New Yorker. Besides my mother being a dominant figure like his mother, I didn't see any similarities that I would call it a made match otherwise. However, both shared that first generation determinism to get ahead, and go for the opportunities that America still offered for the taking and hard work. Neither saw guarantees, as there were few, but both were dedicated to creating better lives for themselves.

Those were the exhortations and expectations bequeathed to me, and their legacy to this day. I want you to know they never told me to become an alcoholic and drug addict, to kill myself or anyone else. My father always said, "Do the right thing," and my mother echoed, "do it." My mother wanted me to graduate from college at all costs and my father wanted me to work. Work being more important than education. Neither really conflicted except they gave me no clear directions, just broad, wholesome directives. What they did do was show me a glimpse of alcohol in their lives, when especially my mother would act silly, fall, and sound senseless, while drinking alcohol. What that did to spur my drinking, I do not know. I recall parties at the house and my mother getting tight, downright intoxicated. When my father drank too much, he always seemed to control himself, become witty and comical, or would just tune out, fall asleep with no acrobatics, no foolish acting out.

I can't recall much discussion about drinking with my parents, beyond watching their drinking behavior. My father however, would comment on my poor conduct when I was intoxicated, and the amount I drank, and said, "You didn't look good. Drank too much and acted foolish." He would remark, "You don't have push, drive, or shove," during my college drinking days, when I didn't progress in a timely or orderly way in school. My mother didn't really say much, other than, I should pay for my own alcohol, and not drink too much of hers. Both tried to keep their drinking out of view from me, not wanting to act indecently in front of me. To them, drinking to excess was acceptable, but not proper. Otherwise not a sin or wrongdoing.

Ironically, my alcoholic maternal uncle suggested I become a doctor. We were walking outside his cloistered small farm one day, when he asked, "What do you want to be when you grow up?" I must have been all of five or six years old at the time when I answered, "I don't know." He then said, "Why don't you become a doctor?" I never forgot his words and from that time on, I was only fixated on doing just that. Do you call that the power of suggestion? I'm not sure what I would call it, but I took it as a command, as I ultimately overcame active alcoholism and drug addiction to be a practicing doctor. My uncle lived a hermit's life working a farm and in a factory. He was odd, drove a motor-cycle, lived with his mother, and never dated women to my knowledge. He always had time for me, and was probably my closet relative while growing up. I have to tell you, he died at a young age of complications of alcoholism and pretty much drank himself to death.

I was also pretty close to a maternal aunt who drank quite heavily. I recall at a young age visiting her and her husband, and how good and alert they looked when I first arrived. Later, his face fell into his plate at dinner, and she began repeating herself loudly, over and over again. Both very nice people, but drunks nonetheless, who died early. Where did I get my wildness when I drank? Mostly from my mother and her brother Stanley.

Stanley was notorious for picking fights when he got intoxicated. Otherwise, he was a really nice man sober. Though he was sick a lot, I am not sure how much alcohol made him sick. He was a farmer who worked on the land and in the factory to support his 10 children. I used to sit on his tractor when he tilled the fields of hay. We'd bail the hay to sell and picked fresh vegetables for dinner. When we were done working in the fields at noon, we would have our biggest meal of the day. I can't say I really I wanted to be a farmer after that experience, but it was really a peaceful time. My uncle died of "heart" causes, as far as I know.

Though my mother drank every day in later life, she lived until 94, failing in her later years. She died of strokes from her heart disease and high blood pressure. Not sure how many more years she would have lasted without damaging effects from alcohol on her heart, and brain.

My father died at 79, before his time. He intentionally stopped taking his heart medications and consequently died of heart failure. He too was drinking daily, mostly vodka, in a depressing assisted nursing home, after his wife died. He probably could have lived more years, as his mother lived until she was 96 years old. I should also mention his wife died of lung cancer from cigarette smoking and alcoholism, at a young age. So I guess my father died of a "broken alcoholic heart."

You ask is there anything I could do to avoid an alcoholic death? Yes. Stop drinking. Studies show that alcoholics die on the average of 15 years prematurely, if drinking alcohol. They can get those years back if they abstain from alcohol for a normal lifespan. Hopefully, that will happen to me, since I don't drink anymore, so that I will not lose years on my life from drinking. I stopped smoking cigarettes too, and the same thing applies to nicotine as to alcohol. Smokers die younger in years unless they stop smoking, and if they do, will have a normal life span.

Maybe I should tell you more about my religious

background to see if you think environment played a role in my addictions. I told you my father was Jewish and mother Catholic. For whatever reasons, I was raised Jewish in my early years, and we actually followed some of the orthodox customs in our home. I also attended Hebrew School to learn to read and speak Hebrew while studying the Torah.

The Torah consists of the foundational narrative of Jewish peoplehood. I didn't know that at the time. I just knew I had to miss playtime after school, was hungry because they never gave snacks, and I had to go three times a week. I never really understood what I read, nor did I speak it particularly well.

I was preparing for my Bar Mitzvah when I turned 13, when I was supposed to become responsible for Jewish ritual law, tradition, and ethics, as well as be able to participate in all areas of Jewish community life. Traditionally, my father was supposed to give thanks to God that he was no longer punished for the child's sins. Of course, my father, who believed in no deity or religion, did not go to synagogue with me. You see his mantra was, "Do as I say, not as I do." I never figured out why his advice was only good for me. I could see in his life where he could have used some of his own advice.

I did not complete my Bar Mitzvah to no one's disappointment, except my father. Instead, I was baptized and confirmed in the Catholic Church at the age of 13. I was certainly as surprised as anyone. The nun who gave me Catholic catechism instructions said later, she didn't think I really got it, and was not sure if Catholicism would stick with me. She was a wise Sister.

What happened is that my parents divorced when I turned 13, my father moved out of the house, and my mother took over officially. Supposedly I was given a choice of either a Jewish Bar Mitzvah or Catholic Baptism and Confirmation. Since I was pretty fed up with both my mother and father, didn't want to read Hebrew after school anymore, and now became the "Man of the House," I chose the Catholic Baptism and Confirmation. I also did not like the outsider life of a Jew in a Christian town and school; I wanted to be popular. Being an identified Catholic was more attractive and expedient. Being a Catholic was still not the pinnacle, but easier to tell my friends than being Jewish.

I continued to practice Catholicism until I hit the wall, and years later realized that Christ was different than Moses, and neither was God to me. What a traumatic experience, but did it drive me to drink? If I only understood life better, and stopped making decisions that were doomed to make me depressed. To this day, I wonder if my religious conflicts didn't contribute to my addictions. Some consider alcoholism a Catholic disease because so many Catholics become alcoholics. And Jews are supposedly immune to alcoholism. As it turns out, I think there are better explanations for my alcoholism and drug addiction.

That explanation lies in genetics. Not too long ago, medical science did studies that confirmed that genetic makeup contributed to who would become an alcoholic, and even drug addicts. The first observations were within families, and concluded that alcoholism ran in families. An alcoholic was more likely than someone without alcoholism to have alcoholic family members.

In my case, I had many members in my family who were alcoholic, my mother, father, aunts, uncles. The next question is why? Was it nature or nurture, genetics or environment, the chicken or the egg? I never lived with my aunts or uncles, but I did live with my mother and father, all were alcoholics. So how could I decide who and what to blame as the cause of my alcoholism?

A doctor I worked for, also an alcoholic, went to Denmark where he accessed adoption records. In Denmark, adoptions were public records, unlike in the U.S. To separate out environment from biological make up, he then compared parents of alcoholic adoptees to nonalcoholic adoptees.

What he found was a major contribution to our understanding of the genetic cause of alcoholism. The alcoholic adoptees had significantly greater probability of having biological parents who were alcoholics than the non-alcoholic adoptees. Biological parents had the genes for alcoholism. Also, whether alcoholic or nonalcoholic adoptees were raised with alcoholic parents or alcoholic environment, did not predict or determine alcoholism in either set of adoptees. His conclusion was that genes were the relevant predictor of alcoholism.

Think about it. Appearances, skin color, height, weight often are similar and determined by genes in family members, and environment has little to do with it, unless someone grows longer legs or has an operation to their change appearance. Environment certainly has effects, but those are more superficial, unless dramatically changed unnaturally. This of course is not a hard and fast rule, nature has considerable variations, and different combinations of genes can express themselves in phenotypes. Which is why maybe not everyone is an alcoholic in a family.

Another clever way alcoholism was shown to be genetic was in what is called twin studies. In these studies, identical twins were compared to non-identical twins to see which was more likely to develop alcoholism. As you might have expected, identical twins were more likely to be concordant or have higher rates where both were alcoholic than the fraternal twins, more than two times, 80% to 40%. What you need to know is that identical twins share 100% DNA, or have the same genes, whereas fraternal twins are really like brothers and sisters, and have 50% same genes. Among twins, genes made a big difference determining disease of alcoholism.

An experienced researcher decided to measure certain responses to alcohol in nonalcoholic offspring. Nonalcoholic sons of alcoholics were compared to alcoholics on tolerance to alcohol and other behavioral measures. The researcher found that the nonalcoholic sons reacted to alcohol similarly to their alcoholic fathers. These alcoholic sons were deemed high-risk individuals to develop alcoholism. Importantly, they showed they handled alcohol like an alcoholic that had not yet developed alcoholism.

By now you must be thinking how much and what genes are responsible for alcoholism. Genes account for about 50 to 60% of the genetic causes of alcoholism. That is significant prediction to not ignore when making a decision to drink alcohol. And if one or more biological parents, is an alcoholic, the son or daughter has at least a 50% chance of developing alcoholism. The genetic influence for alcoholism is the same for men and women. Neither escapes.

We also know that the genes that code for dopamine receptors, a neurotransmitter in the brain, key to addictive use, are identified in developing alcoholism. Addiction to alcohol and drugs appears regulated by genes for cannabinoid receptors, opioid receptors, GABA receptors. Cannabinoid receptors are activated by marijuana, opioid receptors by opioid medications and heroin, GABA receptors by benzodiazepines. Thus, we have a genetic explanation for drug addiction as well as alcoholism. But how do these receptors act to produce addiction?

An important but overlooked explanation is that addiction is a brain disease. Addiction starts and continues in chemical centers in the brain. The main locations are of all places in parts of the brain for unconscious activities like sleep, eating, sex, thirst, the instinctive drive states. That make sense because addiction is an unconscious drive, and is also why conscious control is difficult. Especially if the addictive drive state for drugs and alcohol are associated with basic instinctive drives, as it does. Instinctive drive states express themselves daily, we eat, sleep, think about sex, drink something, reproduce. I like to call drug and alcohol addiction as an aberrant drive state gone crazy. Only in this instance, conscious control is difficult, if not impossible, because the aberrant addictive drive for drugs and alcohol is abnormal, unconscious and uncontrollable. Certainly, I could not control alcohol or drugs at all.

The mesolimbic system is part of the limbic system, the oldest part of the brain in evolution, and represents survival instincts. Dopamine, a neurotransmitter in the midbrain projects to its receptors in the nucleus accumbens in the limbic forebrain. A neurotransmitter is a small chemical that couples with its receptor to cause an effect, in this case to promote addictive use. Increased dopamine is responsible for reinforced, addictive use of drugs. Other receptors are found on dopamine neuronal cell bodies, such as opioids, cannabis (marijuana), to trigger the firing and release of dopamine to stimulate its addictive use.

I like to look at addiction like cancer. Cancerous tissue is uncontrolled growth of cells that eventually overpower and terminate the host. Insanely, the cells eliminate themselves in their destructive drive for replication. Drug addiction is similar as it is uncontrolled use that ultimately destroys its user. Such use is not logical or productive. Neither is addictive use. Or as Humphrey Bogart said, "Play it again, Sam."

> *Every time I look at you I don't understand*
> *Why you let the things you did get so out of hand.*
>
> —"Jesus Christ Superstar" Andrew Lloyd Webber

3

UPPER HALF OF THE BOTTOM THIRD
(Childhood And Adolescence)

"Diogenes was asked what wine he liked best, and he answered, 'Somebody else's.'" —Michel de Montaigne

W ithout even trying, I graduated high school in the top half of the bottom third of my class. I had a D+ or C- average, depending how you categorize a 1.73 out of a 4.0 scale. Those grades are more likely to predict alcoholism, and not medical school. I probably had a learning disability of some kind, and certainly had trouble focusing and paying attention to my teachers and subjects. In elementary school, I remember being carted off to sit in the principal's office so often, because I couldn't sit still or stop talking in classes. One teacher hauled off and smacked me in the face in third grade when I kept talking. She wasn't fair as she placed me in a seat in front of the class within arm's reach. Her aim was too good.

In those days, teachers were heroes if they asserted discipline, and nobody said much. I remember a teacher who had a paddle he used to reinforce order in his classroom, and I was the recipient in a number of instances. No blood, just plenty of smarts. In fifth grade I showed some of my deviant behaviors when I viewed a girl pull down her underwear to expose her pubescent self. Apparently, I knew a lot at the age of 10.

Before that, I remember "playing doctor" with girls as a kid, but just what we did I can only imagine at this point. I did not know bedside manners back then. I was also young for my grade. I really don't remember how all this started anyway. I'm supposing the girls began to expose themselves, and caught my attention, and maybe we talked. I was definitely curious then. I know I wasn't the kind to ask to see, yet I was kind of cute, and not too well behaved, so maybe I stood out to her.

Around that time, I recall an incident when a girl was chasing me on the playground. I looked back for some reason, and when I turned back around my mouth hit the back of someone's head. I chipped a front tooth, but don't remember what happened to the other kid; another example of troubles that lie ahead for me with girls and women. The chipped tooth remains. A reminder to this day, whenever I smile, to keep looking forward.

I really don't remember my grades in elementary school. My mother told me I was so smart that I finished my work in class before everyone else and had trouble sitting still afterwards. Apparently, I got most of my work done correctly. As I understand it, the teachers tried to give me more work to do, but I resisted. Just couldn't concentrate longer to get the required work done. I was already almost a year younger for starting school early for my age, so skipping a grade was not personally a good idea. As I approached puberty, I had an even harder time concentrating and controlling my behaviors, drifting off into daydreaming almost constantly.

I should tell you, I changed many different elementary schools in my early educational life. My father kept switching jobs, neighborhoods, constantly striving to move up social strata, and was just plain restless. As an adult, I vowed my children would not have to do that. With each move, I would have to battle with other kids to assert my place in the school. I was vetted by the school yard bully, not always winning the match, learning how to surrender to the alpha kid.

I think losing was a better way to be accepted than winning, which would create hard feelings. So I'd loose a battle to avoid a war. Besides, I never liked physical battles too much, even though I eventually played contact sports such as basketball, and football. I could endure physical contact as long as I felt in control and did not risk becoming injured. Was I a chicken or good at protecting myself? Probably both.

In 6th grade, I asked my teacher if I could lead the other kids out to recess, as it was customary for a student to do so. I recall her reply vividly to this day, "I wouldn't let you lead ducks to recess." Not a very good confidence builder for sure, and she made her point that I did not fit into her expectations in class. Or maybe she didn't like cute little boys, or kids at all, or was an in bad mood for the day. Who knows, but she was yet another teacher I didn't impress, in a long line of disappointed teachers. An early indicator I would not become a US President. How did I become a doctor then?

So, because I was almost a year younger for my age in school, I was developmentally behind, as you would expect. I was shorter than other kids, and emotionally immature. To this day I think of myself as small and younger, though I am taller and older. Attitudes like that keep me youthful and insubordinate. How much of my early life experiences contributed to my alcoholism and drug addiction? I do not know, nor do I wish to speculate. Certainly, I was maladjusted compared to the average delinquent.

Let me tell you about my shoplifting attempt. I lifted a pocketknife from a drug store without telling anyone, so I outright stole it. Somehow, my mother found it at home and asked me where I got the knife. After some lengthy interrogation, I confessed that I lifted it from the drug store. I am sure I tried to tell her I found it on the street somewhere, but she didn't buy it, and marched me right back to the store to return it and apologize.

The lesson I learned from that was it was not necessarily wrong to steal, but that you can't trust anyone, not even your mother if you commit a wrongdoing. Both parents were high on being "honest and telling the truth." It was another, "Do as I say, not as I do." I'm not saying they were thieves or liars, just that there was lot about the grey lines in life neither told me, even when I asked. Their answer was "little white lies" are ok, especially if the lies didn't hurt you. How do you figure out if they didn't hurt me?

Drugs were not such a big deal in my childhood and adolescence, certainly not as widely used as marijuana, cigarettes, and alcohol now. Instead, I had a mental transformation. Paranoia set in and I had apprehensive fears if I didn't conform to norms. I had to stay away from the bad actors, and that included drugs and alcohol. I became pretty active in the Catholic Church at the time, and was really into principles, morals, and doing good. I started to rely on God, who helped, but also punished. I learned about sin, condemnation, retribution. I had ambitions and thought that the Church would help me reach my goals, stick with the winners and good guys.

I identified with the most popular, liked, and naturally the good students and athletes. Since I possessed little of those qualities through elementary school and middle school, I had a lot to learn and imitate. So I set about making friends with whom had these qualities. I would agree that it was insincere and judgmental, but I wanted to get to the country clubs where all the good, rich guys were. Yet I never quite made it to a country club. I no longer attended Catholic Church, but I did find bad guys and Hell in my addictions.

Because of my natural and acquired drive from my immigrant farm background and Jewish heritage, I worked hard for prestige, status, and success. I wanted to be somebody, a "contender." So I became a social climber, and had no shame in acting and feeling better than myself and others. I thought that's what made you better. Doesn't it? I started dating girls; first whoever would go out with me, then prettier and prettier girls. Usually better students, but that wasn't too hard since I was not very smart in high school. I was more comfortable impressing by being a Catholic than a Jew, besides I never would make it into a country club as a Jew in my neighborhood.

My best friends were WASPs even though I could never be a White Anglo Saxon Protestant myself. Many were excellent students and leaders in the school and good athletes. My best friend was the President of the school in our senior year. On graduation skip day, I rode in the car with all A students. I didn't broadcast I was a D student. You know they didn't ask or seem to care as much as I did. Most of the girls I dated were A students as well. It's not like everyone got D's and C's as I did. I had a special talent for those grades, sitting in class without learning much. That took a certain kind of discipline to sit for years, without any interest in learning.

When it came time to apply for college, I was exposed. My friends were accepted into really good schools,

Ivy league, even! Whereas, I was rejected by all the colleges I applied to and had to use "pull" from my football coach to get into a small Catholic men's college. Otherwise, I would not realize my mother's dream to graduate from college. I should add, 98% of my graduating high school class attended college and I barely made it myself. While I had become pretty judgmental and superficial in my values, most of my friends did not ridicule me.

As for my athletic prowess, my school was "Class B," so not large in size, not a competitive school, and therefore teams had room for me to play. However, I lacked speed. In fact, I was mockingly called Cheetah, due to my slow gait. So I tried out for and made it as a lineman on the football team, a tackle, usually the biggest and slowest player on the team. Admittedly, I was far from spectacular, but played well enough to start on the offensive line. Again, probably too chicken to expose myself in the open field where my lack of speed would get me blindsided by tacklers, but hurt on the more stationary line, I could slug it out with my strength and avoid injury with my quick reflexes. I was smart enough to learn good techniques for moving alongside bigger, dumber players.

Without speed, I played basketball in high school only until I was cut in my junior year. I cried so much afterwards that the coach retracted his dismissal. By then though, I had already been invited to join the wrestling team, which was not as glorious a sport as basketball. Most of my popular, smart friends were on the basketball team. I, however, became a wrestler and overnight got so good that my coach said I could have become a state champion had I come out earlier than my senior year. But, not a status sport.

Nevertheless, I had special pleasure to practice

against the heavyweight wrestler on our team. He was also the tackle I sparred against on the football team. He was an especially nice guy until he got mad, fortunately not too often at me. My first match was against an undefeated wrestler in our league. He was big, strong, and dumb. I recall vividly when he had my back on the mat in a near pin, I heard the music in my head from the movie *Exodus* about freeing the Jewish people. Suddenly, I broke free, and went on to score a victory. Our match was written up in the newspaper and everything. Had I started wrestling earlier, I really do think I would have become a champion like my coach said. Another missed opportunity because of pride and circumstance.

Emphasizing my lack of financial status, I should mention we lived in a very modest, small house, unlike most of my friends. I never wanted anyone to notice, but it didn't seem to matter to my friends where I lived, as much as it did me. I lived with my mother, and my father bought a home close to us so I could visit with him after my parents divorced. I used to spend weekends with him watching football games. I don't recall his drinking too much then, but he was never a talker. He made comments like, "How could he be a champion, when he never won anything?"

Thus, the message was clear I needed to win if I was to be a champion. I had to compete to be the best. Being good was not enough. My father liked renowned colleges, athletic teams. He was a New York Yankee fan, and he thought highly of the University of Michigan, but how would he know? He never graduated from high school.

My mother, on the other hand, knew or cared very little about sports; only sometimes attending my little league baseball games. I started playing at the age of nine, destined to become a major league pitcher. Never saw her watch sporting events outside of that, nor did she attend many of my games in high school. I supplied most of the initiative for participating in athletics. I enjoyed the competition, and thought I was pretty good, but I lacked outstanding athletic ability, and did not really apply myself or receive the instructions to become great at sports. I did acquire the routine of following athletics, professional, college, and high school. I was always interested in the outcome. The score, who won. Big names impressed me. My father read the sports page along with other news daily, and seemed to know what was going on in sports and the world. Curiously, I never saw my mother read a newspaper or magazine, preferring to read popular, romantic paperback novels. She devoured them in batches, yet never talked about them. My father however, I barely saw reading. He watched television most of the time instead. Neither seemed too interested in community or world affairs, and never revealed their political views or candidates or parties they voted for. My father used to say he favored whoever was good for business, my mother would reveal only who she didn't like, but not state the reasons.

I don't recall much debate or discussion about politics or social stories with my parents, though I probably learned my competitiveness from them. To better myself was my single mantra, without much specific direction, other than to not lie and to be sure to graduate from college. I did that with many detours and delays, and as usual, overshot these goals. My father always said to become a professional man, as he himself had wanted to become a lawyer because he could talk so well. He never discussed what other things lawyers did, just that he felt he was persuasive and could make his case as an attorney. A requisite for trial attorneys, he thought.

Unfortunately for him, studying and school were not his passion. He never made it out of high school. I "bettered him" by graduating not only high school, but also college, and medical school. With his regrets, he passed along the poor self-image of males in our family, "No good," according to his mother, according to me. It seemed to me that he did not have much good to say about me either. I recall his comments about how I was not good enough at baseball or football, and always reminded me what I was not. That I would never be much.

My mother was pretty resentful with my father over many things, so I did not grow up with a positive male figure image. Between my mother, grandmother, and aunt, my father could do no right, and was essentially a "bum." Mother's resentments against my father probably still lived on long after she died. The mere mention of his name sent her into tantrums. For sure, I could never say good about him in her presence. Very strange, as he did not return criticism of her. Also strange, was that my father continued to marry alcoholic women, three in fact, before he died. The second died of cirrhosis of the liver, the third of lung cancer from smoking and drinking. My mother became involved with alcoholic men herself, one dying from alcoholic liver disease.

Both parents ultimately chose to drink alcohol, over me and my daughters. After I had quit drinking, I did not want to be around alcohol, understandably, and eventually neither parent wanted to be around us without alcohol. I didn't take it personally, neither did they I don't think. Just shows the power of alcoholism over the choices people make, even in families. Because I didn't witness much drinking in my home growing up, I learned about drinking on my own, naturally. I didn't really pattern my drinking after them. I became an alcoholic without copying too many people. I didn't drink like most of my friends. My degree of loss of control over alcohol stood out early. I was a natural at something, born with drive without willpower.

As you might expect, I did grow up with tensions. I was born into second generation immigrant parents, who were opposites, with no educational or professional history, diametrically opposed religions, Jewish and Catholic, farm versus big city, polarizing sizes even! My mother was 5'3", 120 lbs., my father 6'1½", 300 lbs.; mother good with money, father not. It goes on. Do psychological factors contribute to alcoholism? Does poor self- esteem cause alcoholism, drug addiction? Did my earlier days of behavior and personality problems cause my addictions? Just what is the prevalence of alcoholism, drug addictions, when and how do they start, and why me? According to the Diagnostic and Statistical Manual of Mental Disorders, 5th Edition (DSM-5),

Personality traits or disorders are enduring patterns of perceiving, relating to, and thinking about the environment and oneself that are exhibited in a wide range of social and personal contexts. Only when personality traits are inflexible and maladaptive and cause significant functional impairment or subjective distress do they constitute personality disorders. The essential feature of personality disorder is pattern of inner experience and behavior that deviates markedly from the expectations of the individual's culture and is manifested in cognition, emotions, interpersonal functioning, or impulse control and leads to clinically significant distress or impairment in social, occupational, or other areas of function, pattern is stable and long duration, and its onset can be traced back at least to adolescence or early adulthood.

Importantly what appears to be a personality disorder may be better explained by another mental disorder, effects of drugs and alcohol or another mental condition, or a normal developmental stage, (e.g. adolescence, late life) or the individual's sociocultural environment. When another mental disorder is present, the diagnosis of personality disorder is not made. In my case, did my personality cause my addictions, or did my addictions cause my personality problems? Did I have a personality disorder to explain my pathological use of alcohol and drugs, or did my maladaptive personality cause my addictions? Did my difficulties conforming to social, educational and legal norms arise from my environmental background or my genetic predisposition for alcohol and drug addictions? Did I have antisocial personality disorder before I developed a substance use disorder?

For instance, antisocial personality disorder would look like this: Identity: egocentrism, personal gain, power. Self-direction: goal is personal satisfaction, failure to conform to law or ethical behavior. Empathy: lack of concern for feelings, needs, or suffering of others. Intimacy: Incapacity for mutually intimate relationship, as exploration as the primary means of relating to others, including deceit and coercion, dominance or intimidation. Manipulativeness: to control others, seduction, charm, glibness. Callousness: lack of guilt or remorse, aggression, sadism. Deceitfulness: dishonesty and fraudulence, deceit, fabrication, Hostility: persistent or frequent anger, mean, nasty or vengeful. Risk taking: Engaging in dangerous, risky, behavior without regard for consequences, limitations, denial of danger. Impulsivity: acting on spur of the moment to immediate stimuli, without plan. Irresponsibility: disregard for-failure to honor financial and other obligations or commitments, lack of follow through.

I can't really tell you I developed a personality disorder, though I certainly was not best example of a kid. In addition to being a poor student, I was a behavioral problem in most of life. I later had encounters with law when I started drinking heavily and driving. I was disciplined fairly often for being a disruptive student in school, but not malicious or destructive acts, or fights with students or teachers. You would describe me as attending school but with poor participation and performance in academic achievement. Early on I had trouble forming friendships, particularly, with what would be considered responsible, productive kids. I was an introverted child, spending a lot of time by myself.

My mother bought me a set of drums I played to Bill Haley and the Comets, "Rock Around the Clock." I tried to play the saxophone to copy the current craze in music. I watched a lot of baseball and football on TV. I did not care too much about movies. I did play pick up sports with other kids in the fields and on playgrounds. I did a lot of imagining of being someone other than myself, in another place, doing things I was not capable of. I was a pretty grandiose and unrealistic kid who worshiped athletes, didn't pay much attention to politics or current affairs. Would you call that maladaptive or ambitious or dreaming?

When drinking took off at the age of 19-20, I resembled and became indistinguishable from a personality disorder in many ways. My inner experiences and behaviors certainly deviated from cultural norms. While intoxicated, I showed antisocial behaviors as I got into fights drunk, stopped by police for urinating in public, arrested four times for driving under the influence of alcohol, showing up to work with hangovers. Did I develop low self-esteem, poor self-appraisal, lack of empathy, considerable denial regarding my alcohol and drugs use and their negative impact on others from a personality disorder, or the altering, damaging effects of addictions?

I would call my parents at three o'clock in the morning intoxicated, threatening to kill myself. I certainly showed little concern for them or for myself for that matter. It was doubtful I was intimate in my sexual encounters while in a blackout or under the influence of alcohol; surely without sensitivity. I was egocentric, frequently did not honor my social or work responsibilities by not showing up, or being an drunken ass in social situations, embarrassing myself or anyone else with me.

My mother sent me to a psychiatrist while I was in college who said I was a "rebel," and to me, "without a cause." I can't tell you how many times I drove drunk in a blackout, taking serious risks without regard for consequences to myself or others. I became very callous, lacking guilt, deceitful to myself and others about my drinking and drug use. I wrote checks that bounced, didn't pay my bills. During medical school I always wore the same two shirts and pants, not caring about my appearance as I drank daily and did not see the need to dress in more than a pullover shirt and khaki pants.

The onset of drug and alcohol use in adolescents is typically at age 12-14. The first drug of choice is alcohol followed by nicotine and marijuana. Unlike other adolescents and peers, I did not drink or use drugs until later, when I could prescribe pills. I didn't really drink until I reached age 20 as a sophomore in college, but I became drunk with my early drinking episodes. I had not intended or planned to get drunk; had never experienced alcohol intoxication before my first drunken blackout and fight.

My very first tastes of alcohol were sips of my relatives' beers at a very young age, without much effect. My first glass of alcohol was age 12 when I tried beer from the refrigerator at home, without much effect. The next time I recall drinking was in high school, when I downed a beer or two again, without much effect. Ironically, the classmate I drank with later became an alcoholic and died of cirrhosis of the liver, and I too became an alcoholic and nearly died.

"You don't understand! I could've been a contender. I could've had class and been somebody. Real class. Instead of a bum, let's face it, which is what I am. It was you, Charley."

—*On the Waterfront* (1954), Director Elia Kazan

4

"NO SATISFACTION" AND THE
SEARCH FOR TRUTH
(College Experience, War Years, Philosophy)

"Wisdom comes by disillusionment."
—George Santayana

Here I am in the library in a small Catholic men's college, looking up words in the dictionary, thinking the use of big words is necessary for college work. No offense, but I am in Iowa, in a less than sexy school. The chapel was the biggest building on campus at a college named after a saint I had never heard of, St. Ambrose. To me, Iowa was not the garden spot, but I did manage to be placed in the newer of the only two dormitories. Many of my classmates were from Chicago, similar to me in that this college was their last resort. I was bound and determined to get out of there even if it meant studying and learning! Of course, I didn't know how to study and had never learned too much, but this was the time to try.

I also decided somehow I couldn't get too social or drink alcohol. I didn't know what alcohol did to me yet, but I instinctively wanted to avoid it to achieve success, a foreshadowing of what was to come. For reasons unknown, I had associated alcohol with losers and problems; I wanted to be a winner and succeed. Highly motivated by being in what felt like a monastery to me, I kept praying for God to get me out of there. I kept my religious practices going, attended church, prayed to keep the guilt away, and wanted to get good grades for a chance at another college. I lucked out with a roommate; he was from a farm, quiet, nice, un-assuming, and looked back at me as an oddity for sure. I of course, looked at him as not up to my status. He didn't interfere with me, and I didn't with him, but I certainly was the obnoxious one. Besides, he went home a lot so I was not bothered with social temptations with him, and had plenty of intentionally isolated time to study.

I had few distractions unless I sought them out, and I didn't. It was basically living in the dorm, going to class, eating in the cafeteria, attending daily mass, and studying mostly in my room. Once I got going in classes, strangely I don't remember studying too much, just focusing on my notes, and books. No Internet in those days, so I had to be tempted to walk across campus to the library to read extra books. No computer either, imagine that! I had an electric typewriter, but did most of my work hand written, in script. For the life of me, I taught myself what to do and how to study. I had to get out of that place.

I had my sights set on Notre Dame, believe it or not. I made the trip to South Bend to visit the admis-sions officer to investigate a transfer. By that time, I had collected a large number of recommendations, some from Notre Dame Alumni, for my application file. However, the priest in admissions was not impressed by my D plus or C minus average in high school, and he said to me, "A thick file, means a thick head!" Clearly recommendations at Notre Dame were not weighed heavily in flunkies. But I had not yet accumulated my grade point in at St. Nowhere to impress him. I wasn't sure it would make a difference by his unwelcoming interview, and as it turned out, it didn't. I never was accepted to Notre Dame, probably left on a never-ending wait list. So I chose another college that approved me almost on the spot, the University of Michigan. With new undisclosed trouble ahead.

At St. Nowhere I declared a premedical major towards my dream of becoming a doctor. Thinking whether or not I could handle medical school with my flunking grades, never crossed my mind. I actually started paying attention in class, understanding biology, answering what I thought were easy questions on exams. In German class, the same thing, I understood the discussions and answered the questions correctly. I don't know why, but nothing seemed tricky or hard. My grades were A's, without much of a struggle. My final semesters grades were 4.0 on a 4.0 scale.

I attributed my achievement to not so smart students at St. Nowhere, and not so much my smartness. I carried with me that blind confidence from prior teachers exhorting me to do better. I remembered teachers thought I was smart in grade and high schools, just not good at school work or simply paying attention. I did get a B plus in English, another one of those, "You had too many grammatical errors," just like high school, although the content was good. Now, there I was with a near perfect grade point, looking at colleges to transfer to. I had some reservations as my biology teacher kept saying she had many students accepted to medical school at the University of Iowa from St. Nowhere. I liked her a lot, but St. Nowhere was so far from my identity as "cool," and I had a ticket out.

I had few social contacts or events. I was fixed up with girls at the sister college, St. "Virgins." They were pretty and friendly. We went to bars. I didn't drink. I was practicing chastity and avoiding all sexual contact with women. They seemed unduly disappointed and I seemed not to care. I was not going to get connected to anyone at all costs, I was too determined to escape St. Nowhere.

I didn't interview or apply to places, other than Notre Dame and the University of Michigan. My best friend from high school, a political wizard, introduced me to the Vice President of Finance at the University of Michigan in Ann Arbor at the time. I told him I wanted to transfer to the U-M, and had a good grade point average. My friend convinced me that U-M was a great school, so it didn't take much for me to decide to transfer to there. After my acceptance, I oddly became ill obsessing over if I would decide to stay at St. Nowhere and worrying if I would actually leave. I cloistered myself in my room, except for only classes and meals. But the real changes were religious and emotional. I began to realize that the Catholic faith was about Christ, not just God. I had started my religious life with God. A painful realization to me was that Christ was not my God. I became very depressed and paranoid. Too apprehensive to leave my dormitory.

A deep, dark mood overcame me. I was overwhelmed at the thought of having to go outside of my room except for classes. I stopped talking to people, avoiding almost all personal contact. Frankly, I was afraid that I would be physically harmed. I had been abandoned by my God, and felt very vulnerable to the world. My mood was solemn, lost, bewildered, and disillusioned. I had no rudder, or protection without my religious faith. I had become desperate, I had to get out, I fought any impulse to remain at St. Nowhere, which had become a hostile, frightening place for me.

Soon, I was reincarnated and yearned to fill my dark emptiness. I had left a Catholic college without my God, and landed in a Jewish college, what an allegory! Instead of praying in a Chapel, I was standing on the lawn of the Beta Theta Pi fraternity at the University of Michigan, listening to a rock band, exhorting me to great heights and drunkenness. Now, I had really arrived. Now I was at the mecca, and free from the restraints I had imposed on myself at St. Nowhere. Unbeknownst to me yet, what still followed me was my deep, dark, melancholy, feelings of being lost, abandoned, without meaning or purpose. My God rejected me, was gone. An unacceptable Christ had intruded, and created conflicts I could not resolve. Emerging was the contradiction of my childhood, Judaism vs. Catholicism, Savior–Not-Here-Yet vs. Christ, present everywhere; father against mother, suave city vs. farm.

The answer to my abyss was in the Schwaben Inn, a shabby bar frequented nightly by mostly students, listening to a loud rock band play The Rolling Stones', "(Can't Get No) Satisfaction." A song and title that filled me with purpose. Intermittent bar brawls were sparked by drunken spirits and meaningless crusades. Little did I know just how unsatisfied, and how hopeless and helpless I would become. Day after day I wandered around campus, desolate and purposeless. My mood was black.

I was under the drinking age of 21, but borrowed identification from a fraternity brother for admission to the bars. The checkers at the bar didn't look too hard to keep underaged people out. Soon I became so frequent there, that I was no longer carded. I was such a good customer. I drank a lot from the start, stayed late to close, left in blackouts, not having any sense of what I was doing, guzzling alcohol until I left. Talking about nonsense mostly, not too entertaining, or engaging. I become the person to avoid in a bar.

My drinking began unceremoniously when my new roommate asked if I wanted a drink. I had had little drinking experience to know what to do, while drinking the better part of a fifth of vodka or gin. I just recall a clear liquid containing alcohol. My faint recollection was wrestling with my new roommate, obtaining a noticeable flesh wound in the bridge of my nose. Which left to this day, a telltale scar. With that badge of debacle, you can imagine what stories I made up to explain the first thing someone saw when they met me. Maybe fraternities wouldn't judge me if I explained I was drunk, as that turned out to be a common occurrence in fraternities.

The morning after I hurt all over, even my hair, from a hangover. From the bout. I was terribly sick when I rode my bicycle to the church for Sunday Catholic mass, clinging to the last vestige of hope. You'd think I wouldn't ever try drinking like that again anytime soon, but I did. As it turned out, over and over, repeatedly, and got sicker and sicker. Had I known what I know now, I would have recognized I was an alcoholic from the start, putting together family history, genetic makeup, initial black out drinking, fighting, malignant hangovers, and many, many regrets.

My hopeless gloom continued as I meandered around campus, searching for my God who was dead. I was spiritually lifeless, and emotionally helpless. So, I turned to the study of philosophy, to understand why I felt lost as I did. To unearth what happened to my God or did a God, or I, ever really exist. These were questions I never contemplated before, nor knew existed. Why would I ever doubt I existed, or whether I was mind or matter, being or nothingness, an idea or forms? My introductory philosophy course focused on Plato, as most philosophy courses do, and did not ask many questions about God, not religious based. Still, I discovered questions about reality, if it existed, as well as knowledge, if we could know anything, and what was matter, if it even mattered.

Plato's proof for the existence of God was very simple and straightforward, as he reasoned that most people believed in a God of some sort, therefore, God existed. Otherwise, Plato was mostly interested in knowledge and how we know. He postulated the "forms," as perfect and ultimate truth. We were exposed to the forms sometime early in our existence so we all have a pretty good idea of what is real and true. When you think about it, that makes sense. A ruler that measures 12 inches doesn't measure 12 inches in reality, but something more or less, as no one can make a perfect 12 inch ruler. But most of us would agree 12-inch ruler measures 12 inches in reality, yet ultimately, not really. I was certainly becoming increasingly aware I was not perfect, not even thinking about how perfect I could become.

I buried myself in philosophy courses, and discovered that philosophers argued over the darnest things. An English philosopher, Berkley, posited elegant arguments that matter could be reduced to ideas or mind. When I refer to matter, I mean physical stuff, made up of substance and molecules, like walls we run into. Ideas, on the other hand, are mental products that ultimately matter consists of, and I don't mean mental blocks. Not far fetched from physical theories today that matter can be reduced to mathematical equations.

In a compromise, French philosopher Descartes, decided reality was really both mind and matter, and that mental and physical realities existed. He created the famous proof of our existence for those who doubted it when he said, "I think, therefore I am." Not a bad proof, and hard to refute. And the corollary is, *when I stop thinking, I don't exist, right?* Interestingly, brain death or no conscious viable thought or electrical brain activity is how death is legally defined. Anyway, you wonder how this solved my depression, gave me meaning, and helped to find truth, and lift me out of my abyss? Well it didn't. Are you surprised? I'm not. But it did create ways of thinking I had never considered. In doing so, I expanded my mind to worlds beyond anything I had considered.

Imagine what my fraternity brothers thought when I babbled about mind and matter, forms and truth, God and no God, purpose versus chaos. That's when I was given the name, "Bohunk." Many in the fraternity were given names during "Hell Week," some relevant and others not. Bohunk meant bohemian and philosophical, and probably screwed up and irrelevant too. It also fit the blank, soulful look in my eyes and depressed expression I wore around the fraternity house. And my incessant, nonsensical questions about our existence.

My class attendance dropped precipitously, and wasn't helped by a bridge game that was played more or less continuously throughout the day and night in the main room of the house, near the exit and entrance. Instead of attending class or studying, I made a left turn to the bridge table, and wasted away the day or night playing bridge. When I wasn't drinking, I was certainly living the college life, though not student life.

For those of you who don't play, bridge is card game that takes some mental capacity, and entails bidding for a contract and then seeing if you can make it. It was something I could do with hangovers when I couldn't study. I also didn't have to leave the house to face an overwhelming and perplexing world, as I developed a phobia to class. Classes reminded me how far behind I was. I still have nightmares to this day about not completing assignments. It seems I developed an enduring post-traumatic stress disorder.

I just wasn't up to my game, I couldn't get to first base. I slept through classes, stayed up late at night playing bridge or drinking. The only place I was able to face the world was in bars, and found alcohol helped me stop thinking as I drank into oblivion, blackouts, and stupor. Per Descartes, I could not exist if I got drunk enough to not think, drunk enough to escape my pain.

Which reminds me of another French philosopher, Sartre, who wrote a massively thick book titled, *Being and Nothingness*. Bluntly, "being" was consciousness of ourselves and existence, and "nothingness" was matter or the physical world, outside of our consciousness. Simply, Satre deduced we could know about being, but not nothingness, which remained a mysterious black box. The more intoxicated I became, the more I obliterated my consciousness with alcohol. To be less conscious and more intoxicated was to lose my being; to not exist, and become like nothingness. And nothingness fit me at the time.

My increasing depression and progressing alcoholism created bigger and deeper holes, which, a German philosopher, Friedrich Nietzsche, coined "the abyss." That meant to me a "bottomless depth." You must understand while I was peering over and sinking further into that abyss, I drank more and more alcohol. What I didn't know, is what he later explained, "When you look into an abyss, the abyss also looks into you." I saw emptiness when I looked at myself and looked anywhere else for meaning. Nietzsche foretold what alcohol and later drugs did to me, "That which does not kill us, makes us stronger." And he predicted my later life, "One must still have chaos in oneself to be able to give birth to a dancing star." He made it painfully obvious I did not have a why to explain my state of mind and existence, "He who has a why to live, can bear almost any how." Later, I found my why before it was too late.

What I didn't know is that Nietzsche's searching had the same source as mine. *He who has a why to live can bear almost any how.* Nietzsche himself took huge doses of opium but was still having trouble sleeping. He was writing out his own prescriptions for the sedative chloral hydrate, signing them "Dr. Nietzsche." I did the same thing, and got the same results, near death. He also said Christianity is an antidote to a primal form of nihilism—the despair of meaninglessness. Well, I had lost my antidote. Finding another was one desperate attempt after another, one drink after another, and later bottles of drugs after another, I imagine trying to fill that abyss. Imagine that, Nietzsche was a drug addict, which explained his nihilistic philosophy. He dropped dead suddenly trying to save a horse, imagine that. Do you think drugs were involved? I do.

Our fraternity house was located near a main intersection on campus. I had no excuse not to get to class, which was within easy walking distance. We were also within walking distance of most sororities. We had fraternity parties and invited sororities to our house. We always had tons of alcohol, and loud rocking music. Of course, I got drunk and had blackouts, and wouldn't remember most of the evening, what I said and to whom, when and why. An alcoholic blackout was a regular occurrence for sure, and I don't remember those conversations or events or have memory traces, for a good portion of my college life. It's as if I never lived during those times of intoxication, that were numerous.

One time, a reckless fraternity brother filled the tank

of punch with 90% or 180 proof alcohol, without anyone knowing. You can imagine how wildly drunk I got. I had to be helped into the shower because I was vomiting and delirious. It's a wonder I didn't die of alcohol "poisoning" or overdose that night. I don't know how many fights I started, people I insulted, or really what I did or said. Just another example of my powerlessness of alcohol and life, just another escape from death.

I dated a girl from a prestigious sorority, cute and friendly, and mother like. She invited me to her parents' house for a weekend, and instead I boarded a plane roaring drunk for Grand Bahama. Before leaving for the airport, I shouted in my drunken, grandiose state, in the Pretzel Bell bar I frequented that, "I'm going to the Bahamas!" It must have been around the time of spring break. Sure enough, I woke up on the beach. Not only did I embarrass myself and her, I made a spectacle of myself walking into a casino on Grand Bahama. Full of sand, bearded, in a wrinkled tweed sport coat.

The bouncer looked at me curiously, and didn't exactly throw me out, but I felt so out of place with patrons in tuxedos and gowns. Like a dog with his tail between his legs I soon left when I realized I had no money and no place to stay or eat. I wired someone, either a friend or family, for money to get back home. I don't remember how I paid for the trip there, maybe with another bounced check I was famous for. Back then, we had no credit cards, only a check book. As you can imagine, I bounced a lot of checks. Anyway, I later found out that this girl I jilted was gay. I didn't know that. She is still very nice.

In my quest for truth and knowledge, mixed with alcoholic induced anxiety and depression, I decided to try courses in Psychology. My college at the time was ranked number one in Psychology among Universities. I acclimated quickly to the course work because of my intuitive experiences and it didn't entail much reading or writing. I got to be friends with a graduate student who turned out to be nuttier than I was, but he really tried to help me. I was constantly worried about my intelligence, if I was I smart enough. After all, my grades were not so hot. I was not attending classes, and studying only here and there before I inevitably left for the bar to get hammered with someone, never sure who it might be. Another of my exhorting "there will be no stopping."

Later I'd wake up with hangovers that were not conducive to paying attention in class or concentrating for learning, even if I woke up early enough to make it. I remember I could still handle math classes, mostly because it was an unconscious act for me. I took graduate classes in calculus and statistics. I took logic courses from the master, and survived. I am ashamed to tell you I took the same course in Physics twice, and was very consistent with D's. I just didn't get Mechanics, and barely did better in Electricity. You must be surprised I was still officially a Pre-med major but my average grade point was far from qualifying me for entrance to medical school.

Ultimately, I became a doctor because of the Vietnam War. At the time, my school held many protests on campus, where the far out, anti-war Weathermen originated. Two of my fraternity brothers were Weathermen. Weatherman blew up things as a part of their protests. How do you figure that? We also had All American football players in the same house, along with a varsity gymnast, pre-med, pre-law, and general slackers, like me. And I was usually the house drunk. As Bohunk, I was a psycho philosopher, alcoholic, of gypsy origin, and a person who had informal and unconventional social habits, not unlike an artist or writer. I never saw myself as Bohemian, as I came from a Republican district whose representative eventually became President of the United States, yet I did become a writer later.

I met another philosophy major in the law library where I studied sometimes. He was also pre-med and wanted to become a psychiatrist. A new role model. I also started hanging around with another philosophy major who liked to drink all night and into the next day. And yet another drinking companion was a psychology graduate student who liked to travel and drink, but I don't remember where we went. You had to be smart to get into medical school and graduate school at my University. I had it all figured out; I would become an alcoholic, pilosophical, psychiatrist, physician. And I did.

The U.S. government had other ideas for my future, as it kept taking away my college deferment and reclassifying me 1A for eligibility to be drafted for the Vietnam War. I want you to know that I am not a chicken, and certainly was patriotic. You have to understand my friends were not enlisting, and were deferred for educational reasons... And I kept hearing awful stories about second lieutenants having a life span of 20 seconds in combat. That did not appeal to me, but was a good sign that I still wanted to live, without knowing why. My goal remained to become a wealthy doctor and join a country club. I eventually persuaded my local draft board I was a sincere, aspiring doctor, who wanted to remain a student at Man's Best University. As long as I remained in the medical field in some way, I could avoid the Viet Cong.

During the Vietnam War, President Johnson was always increasing the number of troops deployed, so the pressure to draft young men was ever present. As you know, the war was not popular, did not make a lot of sense to Americans, and did not motivate me to enlist or be drafted, even as an officer. Maybe I knew that I was in no shape, mentally or physically to fight a lethal enemy, especially drunk. I hadn't started to use drugs yet. Marijuana was not yet popular and pills were a thing of the future for me and you.

More trouble, I dated a girl who was pre-med and also wanted to be a psychiatrist, a lovely, kind person. I managed to confuse her with my wayward, drunken ways. She got me fired from my bus boy job in her sorority when we surreptitiously helped ourselves to Cornish hens left over from the meal we missed that day. Somehow, the housemother found out. She wanted me gone because I was dating one of her sorority girls and caused disturbances at mealtime because of my "fraternizing" with sorority sisters. She wasn't the only housemother who deemed me unfit to serve her sorority girls. Eventually, for whatever reason, I slammed a plate down in front of her and was sent on my way.

It seemed I dated girls in every sorority I worked in, as I recall. All were very pretty, and wholesome enough. I presented myself as an ambitious, serious minded, handsome, future something, but hungover. I sort of favored blondes, but I didn't keep that streak going always. To them, I turned out disappointing, with my wanderlust and thoughtless alcoholism. No direction and frequent failures, and not living up to expectations. Talk about frustrations. Always drunk, always drinking away relationships, careers, hope.

My father used to visit me at football games on Saturdays at the university. He would take me out to dinner to watch me get gloriously drunk on martinis. I had dropped out of Man's Best University because I just didn't make it to class and take enough tests. I was in serious academic trouble one semester. My academic advisor wrote on my record, cancel this semester, "To rethink educational goals." He didn't put in, I would completely fail the semester mercifully if I continued. Because I had to be enrolled in a college to maintain a 2S college deferment to avoid the draft for the War, I transferred and enrolled in the Man's *Second* Best University, and managed to stay sober for a couple of months.

I achieved better than average grades, and actually enjoyed my classes. I took English and learned about Ernest Hemingway, who was a drunk and famous writer. Hemingway sought out danger and high risk, fighting in civil wars in Italy and Spain. I identified with his drinking, but not his appetite for war. I got an A in statistics, as my usual fall back in math. Eventually, I decided I had had enough sober education and reapplied and reenrolled in Man's Best University. Of course, almost at once, the drinking resumed in full force. I had learned nothing from my sober time and modest success.

My father one day told me I had, "No push, shove, or drive." I remember that lecture to this day. How could he say that to me, when I was the college man, and he was the high school dropout? You might be surprised that the only person who spoke to me directly about my drinking was my best friend from high school. Shortly after I enrolled in the University, he said, "Norman, you are an alcoholic." Mind you I had been drinking only for 6 months but had just returned from the intoxicated trip to the Bahamas. He had some knowledge of alcoholism, as both his parents were alcoholic. Later, he died of complications of his own alcohol use.

When he told me, I thought he was crazy, and despite failing in school, embarrassing myself in relationships, blacking out at social events, I never gave much thought to quitting alcohol. I just had to figure out how to stay in school and out of war, and on track to where ever I would end up. Anyone's guess at that point. No one was betting on my success or life for that matter. I was not focused on abstinence. My grade point was careening steadily downward but I continued to sell myself as scientist, abandoning philosophy, psychology. I could not get a deferment for graduate school in philosophy or psychology. I could be deferred for graduate school in Microbiology.

An alcoholic blackout affects formation of memory in the temporal lobe of the brain. The hippocampus in the temporal lobe where memory traces originate is extra sensitive to alcohol so that no new memories are formed. Thus, while I had progressed in chronological years, I was actually younger in mental years lived because I did not form complete memories during my alcohol intoxication. Is that why I kept starting over and over again? Is that why I kept failing? Is that why I didn't know why? Because I didn't learn. But I was not done searching.

Addiction propagates alcohol and drug use. A psychiatrist important in the early days of Alcoholics Anonymous, Harry Tiebolt, said the defense mechanisms we use in ordinarily life, are necessary to sustain harmful use in addictive use. Denial, minimization, rationalization of alcohol and drug use, keep the addictive use going and going. Addiction is related to largely unconscious urges, or compulsive drives, similar to eating, drinking or sex, that become attached to or entrained with the drug use. Thus I had powerful instincts that drove me to drink, and later use drugs.

Sigmund Freud postulated the unconscious in his theories of psychoanalysis. His conception of the unconscious basic instincts in the id, and conscience, and sense of right and wrong in the superego. The ego is the conscious mediator of the unconscious id and superego with the world or reality on the outside. Our id controls appetites and sexual instincts, superego generates our guilt and remorse, and together the ego influences and shapes our conscious behaviors.

According to Freud, in order to change our feelings, thoughts and behaviors, we need to retrieve these unconscious experiences to gain control over our appetites. To maintain my drunkenness, I used denial, minimization, rationalization, and projections that kept me unaware or apathetic to the impact of my use on myself and others. I had little conscious purpose in my use of alcohol and drugs, and my unconscious drive to drink was pretty automatic in procurement of alcohol to the exclusion of life, liberty, and the pursuit of happiness.

Addictive use is defined as preoccupation with acquiring, compulsive use, and a pattern of relapse to alcohol and drugs. I certainly spent a great deal of time using alcohol, frequenting bars, drinking at home, eventually prescribing pills to myself. I never kept a large stock of alcohol at home, but regularly purchased alcohol in the liquor store or bars. Although I quit every day almost, swearing off liquor on my way to buy alcohol, promising, "This is the last time!" I said the same thing the next day, and the next day, and the next day...

I didn't think much about the consequences before I drank. I spent a good deal of my stuporous consciousness intoxicated. I exercised little self-control, as I did not have willpower over my addiction. I had a distinct loss of control that led to adverse consequences from compulsive use in every aspect of my life, personal, work, psychological, physical, you name it. My addiction was hard work, with lots of pain and suffering from ill effects. I felt like someone was holding onto me and dragging me up, down, and everywhere. I was on a roller coaster out of control, heading towards crash, after crash.

One day I was walking across the Diag at the University of Michigan, and the terrifying thought overcame me that I could not control my drinking, that it was controlling me, like a train at full speed without a conductor. Evil forces had overcome me. I was no longer the master of my ship, and I was way off course, racing nowhere fast. I was a puppet being forced to do destructive acts to myself and others. Eventually, I was concerned enough to see a doctor in the Student Health Clinic. I told him I thought I drank too much. He examined me and said sure enough, "Your liver is enlarged." He concluded my visit by advising me to cut back on my alcohol intake. That was it, all he said. No treatment advise, no offer of help, no Alcoholics Anonymous, so I was off to another drink, and more horror in store. I was still on the run, not looking back. Medicine did nothing to alter my fatal course. Besides, I learned later that sometimes doctors drink more than patients, and blame patients for what they themselves do drinking.

I can't get no satisfaction
No satisfaction, no satisfaction, no satisfaction

—"(Can't Get No) Satisfaction" The Rolling Stones

5

GRADUATE AND MEDICAL SCHOOLS
(More Alcohol And Pills)

*"He that can't endure the bad will not live
to see the good."* —Jewish Proverb

The draft board was still after me. I had to do something, or face the sure firing squad in Vietnam. But I was more worried that if I dropped out of school, I would never return. My mother constantly affirmed that fear. I had finally graduated from undergraduate college after extending to five years, instead of four, to avoid the draft. One of my continuing regrets is that I didn't invite my parents to my college graduation. Graduation ceremonies for the University of Michigan were held in the Michigan Football Stadium that holds over 100,000 people. The Commencement speaker that year was President Lyndon Johnson, ironically, who almost solely drove the Vietnam War. I felt so ashamed at this point, my grade point was scraping bottom, and I couldn't stay sober much. I had gained weight, was bloated, and didn't feel in a celebratory mood. Mostly I couldn't stay sober long enough to meet and find my way to the Ceremony. I was walking on State Street on campus the time graduation was held; the streets were empty and so was I. I was lost in place I had traveled many times. I had no destination in mind and the present was intolerable.

I decided before graduation to check in with premedical academic counselor. We were talking in an open cubicle surrounded by other waiting students and he was shouting at me, "There is no way you will ever get into medical school, no way." As I walked out, there were many students outside the cubicle staring at me, maybe fearing they would face the same with the counselor. Due to my belligerence, I had caused the line to stack up, because I refused to accept no for an answer. I was deeply wounded, but my drive to enter medical school was not dead. I did not want to admit defeat. Persistence was my lone nemesis and virtue. I was determined to be a doctor drunk or sober. Up to this point, I was drunk far more than sober.

In order to wrangle my way with "pull" into medical school, I started working on research for an eminent scientist, Dr. Levy, who had been at the University Medical Center for decades. His study was aimed at trying to understand effects of localization in response to tissue damage from radiation. I was responsible for injecting tetanus toxin into hind legs of rabbits, measuring response to irradiation or no irradiation.

For the first time, I began to show interest in writing, and helped him with preparing journal articles. He was very appreciative of whatever I could do for him. He was older, but full of energy to work, and the mystery as to why he cared so much, he never explained. I had expressed a desire to attend medical school. However, he suggested I try graduate school, and used his long-standing political influence and stature for me to be admitted to the University of Michigan graduate school in Microbiology. He was a microbiologist himself, and I could continue to do research with him, and take classes.

This meant I had to take some pre-medical courses

that I had delayed, such as organic chemistry, before taking graduate courses. I made extra money that went to buying booze, by working as a graduate teaching assistant in a laboratory for nursing students. I had trouble getting up early enough for the start of the laboratory because of hangovers, and driving a distance from our lake house outside of town. As a result, I also collected a lot of parking tickets and lost my car to my infuriated mother, who took it back.

The perk from teaching the course was I dated one of the nursing students, a pretty, sweet blonde, who I continued seeing after the course ended. With our other friends, we took a trip up north to have an intimate affair, and instead I got drunk and rude. She took off into the woods and tore her ligaments in her knee that required surgery. We drove back to the hospital for her to have surgery. Once again I managed to let alcohol ruin another special occasion for me and someone sweet, undeserving of my boorish behavior.

Dr. Levy moved to Washington D.C. to do research at Howard University College of Medicine under an old friend in the Department of Microbiology. Dr. Levy asked me to go with him to continue his research and look after him. I extracted a promise from him to help me gain acceptance in the medical school in exchange for my continued assistance and devotion. In return, I expected to become a medical student at Howard. We arrived just after the race riots in the District of Columbia, and the atmosphere was tense in the city and medical school.

Howard was a predominately black University, including the medical school. I had never spent much time around black people, and initially did not mix in, out of fear, bias, and prejudice on both sides. To me, I was also not a card carrying or bleeding heart liberal who would show deference demanded in an environment where I am clearly outnumbered and despised among some of the students. But the faculty was professional and understanding. I favored personal responsibility, and given my Jewish background, I was familiar with persecution and prejudice. Up to that point, my solution was to escape into Catholicism, not free of prejudice and not the pinnacle of status, but not as shunned as being a Jew.

I never understood why my Jewish father did not identify strongly with any religious body or conviction. Perhaps he didn't want to get killed, a remnant of the Holocaust, or he wanted to integrate as many first generation of immigrants learned to do. He rarely talked about his battles with prejudice but you could tell he knew his limitations. When he did say something, he recanted his days in New York City when he was chased and beaten by Irish Catholics.

He was pretty big remember, over 6 feet and 300 pounds, so he delivered return firepower. He never acted afraid of anyone or anything, but also looked like he knew the spoken and unspoken rules, and was no campaigner for human rights. He neither advertised nor hid his Jewish heritage, and didn't pretend he was something he wasn't. He didn't think God existed, and before he died he said, "He would be going nowhere, no longer existing in any form or in anyway." He represented or fought for no special causes, volunteered for no missions, and thought hard work would cure all for him.

In many ways he was a typical New Yorker, worldly in the confines of a few square blocks, and always aspiring for greater heights. The journey, not the purpose, was the goal. Yet, he was different than most New Yorkers I knew in he valued fairness more than victory, and in doing things "the right way." He always viewed himself as the little guy, never the big shot, and wasn't much for history or tradition. He was much more likely to demean himself than anyone else. He never talked about his father, and rarely about his mother. He was not particularly educated, having dropped out of school in the 11th grade, and had no college experience. He could tell a joke, and enjoyed a laugh.

For sure, I wouldn't say I was free of prejudice but again I didn't find the black students free of prejudice either. I endured names like "honky," and certainly felt "hate" and "scorn" because I was white. It didn't help that I didn't like it, and was a good student, and naturally had a superiority attitude towards most everyone, not just blacks. I admit, I felt uneasy around "black attitudes" and "black culture" in America. Perhaps a very prejudicial statement I realize, nonetheless blacks without the "patois" and other similar cultural experiences naturally gravitated towards me and likewise. I learned at a young age that speech was a powerful determiner of success, and definer of class and acceptance. In my youth, I made exceptional efforts to learn and use proper grammar and pronunciation, to overcome the "patois" of my parents, immigrant and rural relatives.

A bright oasis in the sea of hostility were the black professors in the College of Medicine. I was totally supported and valued, and never felt discriminated against during my student years by my teachers. I felt respected, but I produced and responded to their efforts and desire to teach, and they were excellent instructors. They were especially focused on learning and certainly current in their knowledge and methods. I was never threatened, nor intimidated. I may have been disliked because of my hungover states, unavoidably arrogant postures, and appreciated for being first in my academic rank in my medical class.

At any rate, I had to take graduate classes for my first year at Howard until I could get on cycle for the next year in the medical class. I entered the Department of Biochemistry, but took Anatomy, a subject I would never grasp. My brain is not wired to trace animate structures and their relationships to each other. I struggled with names of muscles, and neighborhoods of articulations and bones. I could memorize molecular pathways and reactions, that made logical sense. The admissions counselor in the medical school said I had scored well on the MCAT (Medical College Admissions Test), and was admitted despite my mediocre grades.

I was still under pressure from the draft board, and President Johnson kept escalating the Vietnam War. I tried to ignore reading about Second Lieutenants dying by the seconds, as I was likely next in line. So admission to medical school was urgent and my survival, in my mind, depended on it. I did not like physical threats or harm, and war was not for me. Nor did I feel safe in my out of control, intoxicated state. Heavier drinking set in, nightly blackouts, sleeping in, missing classes; with severe, incapacitating hangovers.

I had an appointment with the leading staff member in my U.S. Congressman Gerald Ford's office, to attempt to lobby for research funds for Howard Medical School. I started to shake and tremble while I was talking for the first time. This occasion was before I had discovered Valium for alcoholic tremors, and I was left feeling like a bobble head. I didn't know at the time why, and later experienced frequent shakes in the morning, before a pill or the first drink. I sometimes had trouble holding a glass and pouring liquor, or raising a can of beer until I could establish an alcohol blood level. This sequence continued into my drinking until I took 20 to 60 mg of Valium a day to silence my visible, wired nerves, to work in hospitals until I could reach my next alcohol black out. A later advantage taking opioid pills, was I didn't develop the God awful shakes or feelings of impending doom. Just bottomless depression, suicidal thoughts, and constipation. What a wonderful trade.

I carried a constant sensation of being lost, while trying to get to places I could not reach, and not avoiding places I did not want to reach. My self-inflicted disappointments became indifference and apathy, extolling "this doesn't matter," and my struggle for the next bite of my shit sandwich. I hardly ever planned to get drunk. I just drank, always got drunk, mostly blacked out. On rare nights I didn't black out, I convinced myself I could control my drinking and didn't have a problem. I would write checks in bars, to wake up wondering the amount I spent and covered it later, after it returned bounced.

Frequently, I didn't know how I got home, curious about how I was able to park on the streets of Washington D.C.. Later, I returned to find my car dented, parked oblong after sometimes a long search to find it. I had become immune to peoples' comments, "You are such a different person when you drink," though I didn't recall my conversations most of the time. But I had a strong suspicion I was obnoxious and spoke nonsense, from what little I could remember.

I gradually but surely began to hate myself more and more, sinking lower in a personal nadir of a "batch of wet whale shit." I had endless frustrations at not reaching my goals and changing them to meet my intoxicated level, trumped by my persistent, repeated, senseless bouts of intoxication. The grand question is why I did not stop having goals, and ambitions, as my drinking only increased my naive grandiosity. Because I could not predict my words or actions in my drunkenness, my nameless fears grew and flamed by endless intoxication. And I was having live, waking nightmares about being hunted in the jungles of Vietnam, or on the most dangerous streets in D.C..

When drunk, I sought ridiculous, perilous challenges, only the insane would pursue. I wandered into deep parts of poor, crime laden black sections, near 14th street, looking for prostitutes of all things. Unluckily, a pimp approached me with a gun from my back, and demanded my wallet. As if I fancied myself in a John Wayne movie, I said, "No," to which he responded by firing his gun, lodging a bullet in the back of my leg through to the kneecap. Instantly, I fell to the ground, feeling the heat from the bullet.

To this day, I don't know how I made it to the hospital, I must have driven myself. I was capable of such contradictory acts, to kill and save myself. Believe it or not, it missed arteries, veins, nerves, ligaments, bone. The ER physician merely made a half-inch incision to pluck out the bullet from the top of my kneecap. The interviewing detective on the case couldn't believe its trajectory. Since I was so drunk, I really didn't think much of it.

On another occasion, I found the prostitute upstairs in a room on 14th street, and saw the pimp watching, but he didn't try to kill me this time. He probably found pity with an idiot. Besides, I paid and it was bad for business to harm customers. Surprisingly I could still get it up while so drunk. I don't remember how much I paid, probably all I had in my wallet.

I rented a room not far from the Washington Hilton Hotel on Connecticut Avenue in D.C., in a large house occupied by several men. Some were unemployed, others were students, and inevitably some drunks too. One of my roommates committed suicide after he lost the last sums of money in the stock market. He liked to play the margins and usually lost. He was a graduate of Ivy League and law schools, but couldn't get and stay on track. A thoughtful man, he bequeathed me a six pack of 16 ounce beer, the same brand he drank. I still find it difficult to give him a diagnosis. He taught me the good lesson that the stock market was a lethal and dangerous place. Not that I had any money at the time. I am still not sure how I supported myself back then. My parents rarely inquired about my welfare. Though I would call home for money, cars, and advice I mostly ignored.

Being an otherwise physically healthy male, I had several sexual encounters with women during my stay in that house, some one-night stands, others quite a bit longer. Believe it or not, all nice people. One I met on the street in front of the house. She had a penchant for sleeping with men for free. In college, we called that a nymphomaniac. In my escapades, I never seemed to have a lot of serious conversations, while the outcomes were the same, sex and more sex, never worrying about consequences.

Repeatedly I escaped venereal diseases, pregnancy, and marriage. I was beginning to worry I was sterile because no one became pregnant. As it turned out, I was just lucky. Sometimes I saw them again, most of the time not. I was usually drunk when we were physically intimate, in and out of blackouts. One time I took pity on an older bag lady I met on the street who begged me for money and paid her for a quicky, feeling in a "generous mood." Helping others I thought was not so bad after all.

Eventually, I met someone who wanted me to live with her. I used to walk a roommate's Irish setter in a park not far from my house. I took my customary six-pack of 20 ounce cans of malt liquor to keep blurry eyes on the dog. I usually reached my zenith after four or five cans. Before I got too drunk, I met this cute little blonde who walked her dog too. She looked sad to me, quiet, retiring but had a sexy glow to her rosy, white cheeks. We started to talk, and of course, one conversation led to another that I didn't remember, and I found myself in her apartment one evening. She was anything but a wallflower, she showed me sexual energy I had not quite experienced. I was definitely wanting more, such a sweet embrace.

Her mother and father were alcoholics, and as a child of an alcoholic, I was a magnet for her. She also saw me as medical student to be fascinating, and liked playing doctor with me. I liked her version of medical school and doctoring better. She also wanted to rehabilitate me as she probably wanted to do for her alcoholic parents. I moved in with her, and she gently encouraged me to return to medical school after I had dropped out for a year from drinking.

Miraculously, I stopped drinking. I began feeling healthy, lost weight, started to remember my waking moments, and best of all I woke up in the morning without a hangover. With my newfound sobriety, I made it to class, listened, took notes, studied, learned, and retained vast amounts of medical knowledge. She liked to walk around the apartment nude in the morning, an incentive for me to wake up in time for my classes.

Because I lived on a one-way street off DuPont Avenue, I had to enter from other streets to reach my house. The good news is that meant parking places were available, because people couldn't conveniently reach the street from DuPont Avenue. The bad news is that I ignored the one-way sign when I was drunk. One night I was in my usual belligerent, intoxicated state, and refused to cooperate with police when they stopped me for going the wrong way on the one-way street. The next thing I knew I was in a drunk truck, on cold steel, rolling around on my way to the local jail. I was such a baby when I sobered up, I began crying to them to let me out. A jailor took pity on me, and let me make a phone call to Dr. Levy. He came early in the morning and bailed me out. I think the charges were dismissed because I was a medical student, which worked back then. These were the sort of jackpots I would get myself out of because of my medical status.

Anyway, I forgot to tell you I started medical school on crutches. Although the bullet that penetrated my knee missed vital structures, it still left a great deal of soft tissue damage and swelling. It became stiff and painful after the alcohol and pain medications wore off, and I had to use crutches to ambulate. I recall my first day of medical school, I stood at the back of the amphitheater, on my crutches, listening to an Anatomist explain most of the height in humans was in their legs, and sat a short and tall person next to each other on a table to prove his point. Their heads were at equal height sitting down but not standing up. I especially recall the demonstration because I couldn't stand long on my exquisitely sore, wounded knee. But I attended classes until I could discard the crutches. Lucky again, the pimp knew to shoot me in the left leg mercifully so I could still drive, using my right leg. I will never know if he intentionally aimed at the left and he was a marksman and was such a terrific shot to save my leg from amputation. I'm not sure if I really told anyone what really happened, rather explained I had twisted my knee playing volleyball. Though I did play volleyball, while drunk, I never twisted my knee from it.

As I limped into medical school from jail so to speak, I quickly gained an unstated reputation as a drunk.

I was told I was misunderstood instead. By this time I had beaten the draft board by entering medical school, and subsequently Nixon ended the Vietnam War. I was no longer subjected to the impending kidnapping by the draft board. Instead, I was having trouble staying out of jail, shootings, and hospitals. I am not sure why I thought Vietnam was not safer; at least there I had an enemy other than myself to fight. Further, I could blame my defeats on the Viet Cong and President Johnson. Finally, Johnson told the country, "I will not seek the nomination for the Presidency of the United States," to the delight of many, since his war policies had torn the country apart. Personally, I certainly was glad to see him go. I was tired of running from the Viet Cong thousands of miles away, and rather chose to dodge bullets and spend time in jails at home.

I used to think alcoholics were old men in trench coats who lived on park benches, and drank liquor in brown bags to disguise their obvious intoxication. I never imagined I could become an alcoholic, because that identity didn't meet my expectations. Little did I realize, my denial would never allow me to see myself as I really was: a young version of the drunken bum. Unbeknownst to me, I was a chronic alcoholic dressed in the veneer of respectability of college and now medical school. While I had fits and starts, ups and downs, I managed to progress enough to move from one log to the next, rolling and falling but not completely drowning in my sea of alcoholism.

The average age of onset of alcohol dependence in the U.S. is 22 years old for men and 24 years old for women. That means half of those who become alcoholics do so in their early to mid-twenties. Many are alcoholics as teenagers, and even younger today. Alcohol is frequently the first drug used, followed by nicotine, marijuana, and other drugs. Today's alcoholic, as I became, is addicted to and uses multiple drugs. While drinking, I smoked two packs of cigarettes a day. Both my parents smoked cigarettes, and after having headaches from their dirty habit, I swore I would never smoke. I never caught on to marijuana but that was more of age thing then, and marijuana smokers were younger. Later, I did get hooked on narcotics and tranquilizers, when I could prescribe to myself.

Paradoxically, I was usually depressed when I drank, and not depressed when I could abstain from alcohol. Yet I relapsed to alcohol. The debate rages on whether it is the chicken or the egg, and if alcohol causes depression or is a medicine for depression. Alcoholics frequently rationalize their drinking by complaining they drink because they are depressed, and remain depressed while they drink. Because alcohol is a depressant, their depression, however, significantly lifts when they sober up.

In a study done years ago, a Harvard researcher examined the psychodynamics of alcohol intoxication. They entered known alcoholics into a study, and noted their anxiety and depression were normal before giving them alcohol. When alcoholics were asked why they drank, they maintained because they were anxious and depressed. As they drank more, and became increasingly intoxicated, depression set in and increased with continued alcoholic consumption. Some became suicidal. After they were detoxified, their anxiety and depression resolved abstinent alcohol. Curiously, when asked again why they drank, the alcoholics responded because they were anxious and depressed. Alcohol as a so-called self-medication, worsens the depression, does not make it better. The alcoholic mind plays tricks on them, and deludes into thinking alcohol helps depression and impairs their insight and judgment for realizing it is depressing. I like to think of it as a delusion that kills, as some delusions do.

Sex is normal, right. We spend a lot of time thinking about sex in many ways. How many times during the day do we stare at bodily anatomy and daydream about sexual fantasies, undressing and caressing. Also, more and more spend hours viewing pornography, a newer expression of sexual outlets, and even addictive behaviors. Sexual instincts are strong and expressed in so many ways personally and socially. Almost anything is sold with sexual implications. Alcohol for some releases sexual energy and disinhibits sexual impulses for others. Alcohol is an aphrodisiac in moderate amounts and fuel for aggression in larger amounts. Desire for sexual gratification accompanies alcohol intoxication, impairing judgment, opening the gate for sexual desires and consummating in the sexual acts. Frank aggression is an unfortunate outcome in some intoxicated individuals. However, alcohol can interfere with intimacy and sexual performance, such as erection, ejaculation, and orgasm for both men and women.

Early on, I experienced sexual energy and enhanced performance when I drank, but lost sexual interest and performance in later years. My sex drive and performance further deteriorated on sexually incapacitating drugs, such as narcotics and tranquilizers. Sexual behavior can be viewed in men and women as desire or arousal, erection or stimulation, ejaculation or orgasm. Men and women have similar sexual anatomy and physiology, and both respond to sexual stimulation. Interestingly, women have shorter refractory periods between orgasms than men, and are capable of multiple orgasms. Alcohol and drugs interfere with all stages, and provokes aggressive behaviors. According to Freud, sex and aggression occur together in the id. Alcohol can provoke both. Combined with poor judgment and delirium, it can be a recipe for conflict and violence, at least hurt, victim-like feelings. Impotence is lack of sexual desire or performance, and is common in both alcoholic men and women.

Because alcohol addiction is related to sexual instincts, sexual addiction occurs in alcoholics. Sexual addiction is a preoccupation with acquiring sexual objects and excitement, compulsive use of sexual stimulation, and a recurring pattern of sexual acting out. Excessive masturbation and pornography are examples of compulsive, addictive sexual activity. Hours can be spent on the Internet, viewing explicit, graphic, sexual activity. In person, sexual acting out with varying partners is another possible example of sexual addictive behavior, either in the intoxicated or sober state. Sexual activity may actually increase in the sober state, as an addiction can replace another addiction, and sex can replace drinking. Any gender can engage in sexual addiction, with opposite or same sexes. Adverse consequences accrue from sexually transmitted diseases, unplanned pregnancy, rape, infidelity, and you can imagine the rest. I didn't realize I was becoming an expert in another addiction. Later about my sex addiction...

Take a look in the mirror and cry
Lord, what you're doing to me

—"Somebody to Love" Jefferson Airplane

6

THE GREAT ESCAPE (Residency)

"Never let the fear of striking out get in your way."
—George Herman "Babe" Ruth

As an alcoholic, I continued to drink. After I had a period away from alcohol, became comfortable living with my girlfriend, was excelling in school, and feeling good, inexplicably I returned to alcohol and my misery. My first two years of medical school were drunk or sober, largely buried in books, memorizing and learning pathways, diseases, medications. I had to be conscious and alert to retain piles of textbooks, and apply information to exams. But now came my clinical years, and more drinking, even on the job. Failure had become a common theme for me. I could not keep from drinking, nor could I respect myself. I struck out when it came to drinking, time after time. Though I was not a baseball star, I became an alcoholic, just like Babe Ruth. He died young, but here I am, still swinging. He hit more home runs and struck out more than any player, and drank through his baseball career.

Here I was in medical school finally, but still drunk. Though a lower ranked school, I learned that if I performed well academically, I could get a residency at a prestigious place, and launch my career in medicine. No doubt I took long enough to get there; many drunken detours, and not too many roads not taken in my quest for success. Even in my intoxicated state I ventured into many areas due to my curiosity, and little interest yet in a destination. You can imagine I was living in a philosophical fantasy, fueled by alcohol and pills. A dream world of not too many don'ts and too many do's. Not too many applauding.

On my ultimate, suicidal trip to the Intensive Care Unit, I had many starts and stops due to alcohol and drugs. I managed to finish high in my class my first year in medical school, but I was focused on doing well on national boards for licensing, called Step Exams in those days. If I scored high, doors at residencies would open up as they still do. However, this was a national competition. I would be competing against medical students in all medical schools, not just those at Howard. Right or wrong, national exams are the ultimate measuring stick for medical graduates. I knew I wasn't dumb, at least I hoped not, but I had previously spotty academic success on standardized exams. There was little reason to believe, based on performance, that I could excel in medicine, let alone on a national level.

In grade school, I could have been diagnosed as having attention deficit disorder. I was thrown out of many classes for not paying attention, and had so much trouble focusing on and attending to academic work or social interactions. I hardly ever got good grades in my schoolwork or even citizenship. Because I bugged the teacher so much, and other classmates, because didn't follow directions. Anyway, I could never understand what teachers were trying to tell me. I could only listen for a few minutes, and then wander off into Never Never Land. I could not follow teachers' thoughts through to conclusion. You can imagine why I didn't listen, if I couldn't listen, and why I didn't care about what they said, if I couldn't care.

My early testing days were not promising to be

admitted to a medical school, forget college. It turned out I was later rejected by most colleges, because my high school grades matched my SAT scores. My SAT scores in high school for college admission were average in Math but quite low in English. I attributed that to my absence of role models in speech, my immigrant background, poor performance in class, and probably a learning disability. Also a speech impediment. I was stutterer. Math was something that didn't necessarily require much learning, just native ability to abstract concepts and numbers, whereas English was based on usage, learning and cultural practice.

Honestly, I was too drunk to remember my MCAT scores for medical school admission, but they were based some on acquired knowledge, though intelligence is a big factor. As I said, my admissions counselor in medical school commented that my MCAT scores were quite good, that probably reflected my academic experience in college and whatever native intelligence I didn't drown in alcohol. All I remember about my MCAT score when I opened up the envelope, is that it didn't meet my expectations, and I got gloriously drunk. But I didn't take the time to review the scores carefully, and then again, I never met my expectations drunk or sober, nor especially my Dad's.

What I could not explain is that drunk or sober, I was able to learn medical school material. After years of study and eventual practice in Neurology and Psychiatry, I determined I had an immature brain, that took longer than most to mature. In humans, encephalization or brain growth correlates with brain maturity, and brain development proceeds at different rates in people, slower in males than females.

I doubt alcohol helped my brain development, but I don't think it slowed or sped it up, it did that on its own. Another famous baseball player, Mickey Mantle, who played for the Yankees said, "Sometimes I think if I had the same body and the same natural ability, and someone else's brain, who knows how good a player I might have been." Well I didn't have someone else's brain, and I had to wait for it to catch up to my body and ambitions. I had a disconnect between my goals, my aspirations, and my brain. Babies born prematurely lack encephalization for their body size, and it takes time for the brain to catch up. Mickey Mantle was an alcoholic most of his baseball career, set batting records, was known as a carouser too, and died of alcoholic cirrhosis of the liver.

Despite his playing with an alcoholic brain, he said, "Somebody once asked me if I ever went up to the plate trying to hit a home run. I said, "Sure, every time." So it was with me, I always tried hitting home runs, never satisfied with a base hit, always going for the fences. At some point in my mid 20's, my brain caught up with my body, and I started to learn and understand, and importantly pay attention. Medical knowledge started coming easily and I worked at improving my understanding. I even started deriving pleasure from learning, and best of all could apply it at least to tests, and later clinical situations. But I stayed drunk, and later drugged most of the time.

Anyway, I took Part I of the National Board of Examination (NBE) and surprisingly to me, I scored in the top 10% overall among U.S. medical students. My score in anatomy pulled me down, but my score in Pharmacology raised it. In Pharmacology I obtained a near perfect mark. That foretold my future, and also reflected my preoccupation with drugs at the time. Whenever I applied my medical knowledge from my personal use and experience with drugs, it was for worse than better. But my scores set the stage for the great escapes, as I was able to move from residency to residency sometime before I fell through the floor, or was captured during my alcohol and drug use.

I had applied for a list of residencies that included big, famous and prestigious medical centers and universities. I listed a Harvard hospital first, the University of Chicago second, and the University of Michigan third, and I placed with U-M. I remember Howard announced student matches in an auditorium and I groaned when mine was was called out. Now I was returning to familiar territory, a scene of heavy drinking, and not a new, exciting adventure or escape. But it was prestigious, ranking in the top 10 medical centers, and I had reached a new zenith, at least I thought. How little I knew how unprepared I was to meet the rigors of a challenging internship in internal medicine. Of course, Dr. Levy had greased the wheels with his recommendations and my rank of second in my class at Howard, with the top NBE scores in the school and high scores in the country, pushing me over the top.

When I mean I was not prepared, I mean I was *not prepared.* You see while I had studied for the preclinical years, basic science courses such anatomy, biochemistry, microbiology, pharmacology, pathology, I did not take my clinical rotations as seriously. My drinking resumed as I had more time and much less interest in clinical medicine than basic science; I blew off clinical rotations. I recall my first rotation in obstetrics and gynecology, and being woken up at three in the morning with a hangover to stand over an about to deliver mother in a cold, bright room filled with steel and sheets. I felt totally inept and had no sense of the next steps or what to do. When asked to perform a neurological evaluation of an obstetrical patient, I started with cranial nerve, which is for smell. You need to know, no student, resident or neurologist starts with an examination of smell. And I used a stimulus that was irritating and did not accurately assess smell. Not off to a good start. No clinical sense, for sure.

I could not tell you what was important in a history or examination. I did not grasp dilation and effacement of cervix in anticipating woman's readiness for delivering a baby. And why listen to fetal heart tones, what did they tell me? I always heard them loudly and clearly with the amplified monitor. The worst part was trying to grab the slippery infant as it squeezed through the pubic opening, worrying about dropping it in the middle of the night. I could never remember whether to raise or lower the baby attached to the umbilical cord, to avoid draining blood back to the mother. It never seemed to matter at what level the baby was held, it always had enough blood. Then I fumbled with where to clamp the umbilical cord before severing it, to finally separate, once and for all, the baby's connection from the mother physically. I couldn't wait to hand the baby to the nurse, and get this worry off my hands. I mostly felt anxious during the birth, didn't appreciate the experience.

I forgot to mention, most mothers screamed bloody murder during the delivery, which didn't make my mood any better. I couldn't figure out why modern medicine was so barbaric when it came to birth. Mothers looked anything but joyful, were exhausted, and horrified at the whole event. Perhaps due to my first experience in Obstetrics, I spent future nights in the call room drinking. I would sneak out to a liquor store, buy beer, bring it back to the call room and get drunk. I don't know if I was called or not because I slept like a corpse in a tomb when I was drunk, and couldn't hear the phone. Maybe the attending physician didn't want to bother with a medical student slowing them down. Anyway, luck or not, I never had to show up intoxicated in the delivery room.

I do have to put in a deserved plug for the Chair in the OB-Gyn Department. His lectures were among very best, mostly, physiological and endocrinological explanations of pregnancy, menstruation, fertilization, and gestation. He was a fascinating and inspiring teacher who made a lasting impression on my career, even if I didn't care for the clinical part.

Next rotation was medicine at old Feedman's Hospital. We saw patients in large wards, not unlike other hospitals at the time. The Department of Medicine had a famous Chairman who was Howard's equivalent to William Osler from Johns Hopkins as a mythical figure in medicine. He was a humble, dignified man. However, I was left uninspired by my experience in clinical medicine. I got lost in taking long histories and doing physical exams. I could never get the big picture, and put the history and physical together into a clinical disease. I didn't really practice and improve my clinical skills, learn how to take an Electrocardiogram, read X-rays, draw blood, start IVs, and monitor patients for clinical signs and symptoms. I just seemed to wander from patient to patient, confused as to what to ask, bored to death with idea of being a doctor, if this is what I had to do, time after time.

You can see I was not ready for the grind and gruel of the internship at Man's best hospital that lie ahead. I was totally oblivious to what was next. I had always somehow survived the worst, and I had just finished best in my class to my way of thinking. Besides, I understood medicine. I had a marvelous pathology teacher at Howard who left me with an indelible and unforgettable understanding of basic diseases, inflammation, immunology, heart disease, cancer. What more did I need to make it at my next stop?

My graduation was another waste. I did attend with a large tumbler of gin, and don't remember much from a blackout; just as I had given the lead speech for my Alpha Omega Alpha Medical Honor Society, in an alcohol blackout. AOA represent students who finished in the top ten percent of the class. I had been chosen to give the speech, was told I was misunderstood. A surgeon had selected me to give the talk. He didn't know I was a drunk. He came up to me afterwards, and said I had done a good job. For some reason, surgeons liked me and I liked them. We resonated. They had commanding personality and acted like heroes. Another fantasy I carry today. Beyond personality, I have little in common with surgeons. I don't like standing so long in operating rooms, and wouldn't dare to make cuts so high risk.

What I didn't consider as I packed my car to leave the pretty blonde and Howard, is that I would leave lifelines of support. Up to that point, I had not yet tried to kill myself, been admitted to a hospital, arrested, or gotten into serious trouble with my drinking besides destroying a relationship. Dorothy, had been my pillar of support. She literally held me together, piece by piece. She was the glue. She tolerated my drinking privately. I used to walk her dog at night and buy beer, and hide it outside or inside apartment. I drank a lot of warm beer in the summer. No matter, I just wanted the alcohol. I snored a lot, and she never complained. She was looking forward to graduation but I wasn't. I was returning to my land of defeat. I don't know what possessed me. I had met her with sexual excitement and satisfaction, and was now leaving her without sexual response and in no satisfaction. I had rendered her frigid emotionally and sexually with my daily drinking, with my aloofness and callous self centered pursuit of alcohol.

Just like her parents, she was not able to stop or cure my alcoholism. We defeated her, as I saw her crying and waving in my rear view mirror. I did visit her years later when I was still drinking, and I couldn't bring myself to sexually or emotionally hurt her again. I shouldn't have seen her. So, I decided as I returned to the bar to guzzle more scotch or gin, whichever kind of alcohol it certainly was, I had become such a terrible person.

The terror continued. My first rotation was on the Pulmonary Intensive Care Unit. I had to be up all night, and the service had the reputation of having the sickest patients in the hospital, with end stage lung disease, unable to breathe unassisted, without ventilators and medications. It was probably the most demanding personally and professionally, especially for an intern, and I was completely unprepared to take care of dying, breathless patients. Highly trained nurses wrote my intravenous fluid and medication orders. I had a respiratory therapist who wrote my ventilation and medication orders. All I had to do was show up, but I couldn't even do that.

The biggest problem being I was unaccustomed to working 36 hours straight without sleep. I'd go home and get drunk, and wake up in time to report by 8 am. I remember getting calls from residents who were first concerned and then irritated by my blatant, irresponsible approach to my internship. I can tell you that I became delirious from holing up in a confined ICU that had lights on 24 hours a day, machine pumping lungs continuously, patients who could barely move, much less talk, myself in serious alcohol withdrawal, in and out of intoxication, severely sleep deprived, completely confused and lost, lost.

Surprisingly, I should have mentioned up to this time that no one had suggested treatment for my alcoholism, and I don't recall anyone ever mentioning Alcoholics Anonymous. Rarely did anyone even discuss my drinking, and I certainly was not asking anyone to do so. Despite being the drinker, and the drunken rummy, I was the last person on earth that wanted to do anything to help me stop drinking. I smoked cigarettes back then, and one night I fell asleep on my couch and set it on fire. The smoke woke me up somehow, and instead of calling the fire department, I picked up the burning couch and threw it out the balcony in flames onto the front yard. I went back to sleep and discovered it smoldering in the morning on my way to the hospital. Didn't think much more about it, just another drinking debacle, I soon forgot. Didn't everyone fall asleep to flames, drunk?

I remember choosing my apartment because it was located near a bar I frequented on my way home from the hospital. I hadn't been stopped yet in Ann Arbor for drinking while driving, but it wouldn't be long. On my way to or from somewhere, I got lost on a city street. Ann Arbor streets had changed since I was an undergraduate student, so I naturally wove over curbs and medians due to unfamiliarity and a blood alcohol level of .22 when the police arrested me. I woke up in front of the judge and made the excuse I had to report to the hospital as a medical intern. Frankly, I can't remember if he bought that story or not.

Before the DUI (Driving Under the Influence) wound itself through the court, I got another one. This time it was with a friend from undergraduate times who was practicing medicine, a fine fellow, who drank as I did. I woke up yet another time in jail and charged with a DUI. Before the print dried on the second charge, I got arrested for standing next to my car in an intoxicated state, a charge I thought was grossly unfair since I wasn't driving. Guess what, another DUI charge for my fourth in six months, and just over half way through my internship.

To say I was in a pickle would be more than minimizing my circumstances. Fortunately, and unbelievably, I had not yet caused an accident. (More to come). I am not sure if I even had attorney yet before a mysterious doctor showed up at my doorstep, literally. I think my Department Chair notified him about me. He said he worked for an alcohol treatment center in Brighton Michigan, near Ann Arbor. Further explaining he could make a deal with the court, if I entered treatment for my alcoholism and fulfilled community service. If I complied, the judge would dismiss my 4 DUI charges, and my Department Chair said I could return to my internship without prejudice. I can't recall if jail or prison time was the alternative but I didn't want to find out.

So I went, and spent not quite 2 weeks in inpatient alcohol treatment. I met another doctor who detoxified me who said, "You are powerless over alcohol, so you drink," inferring that I didn't quite get the idea of abstaining from alcohol. He was right. I was not ready to quit drinking yet, and I don't know why; a mystery to me. What more did I need to know, experience, lose, gain, from continued drinking?

I did hear something that eventually saved my life and gave me a much different way of living. In treatment, I had attended AA meetings, and learned that when, and if, I decided to quit drinking, AA could help me. I remembered AA members who looked differently than I felt, and appeared released from that God-awful compulsion to drink. I recall listening intently to the "primary purpose" read by a very clean looking, confident man:

> Alcoholics Anonymous is a fellowship of men and women who share their experience, strength, and hope with each other that they may solve their common problem and help others to recover from alcoholism.

The only requirement for membership is a desire to stop drinking. There are no dues or fees for AA membership: we are self-supporting through our own contributions. AA is not allied with any sect, denominations, politics, organization or institution; does not wish to engage in any controversy: neither endorses nor opposes any causes. Our primary purpose, is to stay sober and help other alcoholics to achieve sobriety.

Well I will set you straight right here and now, I did not have a desire to stop drinking. So that's that. I wanted nothing to do with sober alcoholics, in or outside AA, period. No way, over and out. Just why, is still a mystery to me to this day. I do know I had a God-awful fear to live without alcohol, and I could not face life without alcohol. What if I couldn't accomplish my plans and goals sober? I truly believed I was more likely to succeed drunk and disorderly. I'd bet my life on it. Is that insane?

I decided Ann Arbor was my problem, not my drinking. Also, I drank because of the stress of a medical internship, sleepless nights, clinical decisions, life and death stakes. Why not try pathology, no live patient care, intellectual explanation for death, slow pace, and I could drink. I should add, I had found pills helped me tolerate the stress of my internship, as I could down propoxyphene, a narcotic opioid drug, while I worked, could borrow some while on duty, or prescribe for myself. I discovered I didn't need as much alcohol to stay intoxicated, didn't get arrested as much, and could wake up in the morning to report to work. I didn't study often after I graduated from medical school anyway, so I didn't have to think. I had become so good at faking it, so good I believed it.

Naturally, when I started my pathology residency at the University of Chicago, I had to continue to treat my ills with pills, and I started experimenting with different types of drugs. I found that the pills energized me, instead of putting me to sleep and dulling me as alcohol did. I tried codeine because so many doctors prescribed it for pain or whatever. Someone suggested chloral hydate for sleep, or a Mickey Finn with alcohol. Somehow, I read that another sedative, placidly, was not addicting. And I still kept drinking, so I was mixing pills with alcohol, a lethal combination.

By this time, I was unable to moderate my drinking at all. I would hang sheets over my apartment windows, so I would not know if it was day or night. Especially day, as I could not stand the daylight at this juncture. I took the phone off the hook and drank around the clock, leaving only to resupply alcohol and pills. I can't tell you how many weeks I kept up this routine, and what I told the pathology department. I think I may have called in sick at some point, but how often and what excuses I used, I don't recall. It was one of my most prolonged binges, and darkest bouts with alcohol and pills. I honestly don't think I actively thought of suicide, but I don't think I put up much of a fight to live.

For whatever reason, I passed out near the door of my apartment into the hallway, and had left a crack open. I think the pills were the culprits, and I didn't mean to park there for the night. The next thing I knew, I woke up in a literal straight jacket because I had become so wild at the Emergency Department, in the University of Chicago. The same place I was a resident. I realized I had woken up in the Psychiatry Unit, already trying to figure out how I was going to get myself out of here. Again, I gave little thought to how or why I ended up in a straight jacket on psych ward. No, instead all my energy was devoted to getting out of this yet another jackpot. Just another incidental jam, passing out in the wrong place so someone could find me.

My answer to this embarrassing exposure in a hospital where I was a resident, was to transfer to UCLA in Los Angeles. So my mother and I drove from Chicago to L.A. in time to start my university residency in clinical pathology. You see, I always had an escape plan for my next flight from reality. The residency did not interfere much with my drinking or drugging. But I was terrified to drink and drive on the freeways in L.A., so I drank in the apartment, or walked to bars in Westwood.

I managed to bring some nice looking girls home with me in my drunken pleasure. I began waking up with strange women even though I had stopped driving. One woman followed me from Chicago; I had fooled around with her in my apartment there. We had gotten complaints from neighbors who saw us naked in the living room doing whatever we were doing. I still remember her tan line from the California sun. She was a bit crazy, even for me, but I accommodated her after she unexpectedly visited me from Chicago. I am not sure how many other women, as my memory at this point was fading fast, as the combination of pills and alcohol were erasing so many experiences.

I was out of ideas. Here I was caged in this beautiful apartment in Los Angeles, afraid to leave for fear of incarceration or death. I had rented an apartment within walking distance of the UCLA medical center. I sensed just how out of control I kept becoming, and had no idea where and why I was running. I continued to swallow pills and alcohol without hope. I just couldn't keep from taking the next pill or drink. In one of my rare moments, I asked Christ for help with my drug and alcohol problem. I was standing when I cried out. Nothing happened. Just then anyway. I wouldn't ask again for a long, long time.

The pleasant, warm, sunny, cloudless days began to

bug me. I scoured the sky for clouds, darkness, rain, to match my desolate mood, but nothing. I had been thinking about psychiatry at this point, between the bottles of pills. I was still able to prescribe for myself at the medical center. I had made connections with faculty at UCLA. So I just left, not sure I told anyone why. I decided to go back home to the Midwest where I could drink more safely, I thought. I felt at the edge of the universe in LA, more out of control than usual.

After returning to the midwest, I met another lovely woman, considerably older than I was. I told her I was an alcoholic and had lots of trouble with alcohol. I had started attending AA, but could not make a connection. To this day I don't know why, I just couldn't. I was looking for ways to moderate or fix my drinking problem by myself. It was Jennifer. She said, "Try me instead of AA." It didn't take me long to decide which I would chose. I also had signed up for a residency position in my hometown at Michigan State University. That lasted for two months. I walked out without so much as a goodbye. I was out of explanations. My cure was death. So I thought, as I headed to Man's Best Hospital.

Wipin' out wipe out
Wah wah wah

—"Wipe Out" The Beach Boys

7

"HOPE SPRINGS ETERNAL"

"Hope is a waking dream." —Aristotle

When I applied for residency positions in Psychiatry, I had received a call from Johns Hopkins about an opening. I traveled to Baltimore, Maryland to interview. I decided to move in with Jennifer and begin a residency at Man's Best Hospital. I was in full bloom, alcohol, pills, marriage; running as far from help as I could. I had been in 5 residencies in less than 3 years. I was running on gas I had accumulated in medical school, top grades, high test scores, and residency tours, though brief, at prestigious programs. I kept landing in the best spots though crippled by drugs and alcohol. I had developed a whopping narcotic addiction in five states and residencies programs aided and abetted by being a physician and having access to pills through self-prescribing.

It was in medical school when I first encountered pills. I had become close to a mentor at Howard who specialized in Endocrinology. We discussed many topics in medicine. I was having new problems with premature ejaculation. You can imagine how important that could be, so I asked my professor about it. He suggested I try Valium. Of course I didn't tell him I had resumed drinking alcohol. And he didn't tell me Valium was addicting. After I sobered up, I learned that alcohol withdrawal induced premature ejaculation due to heightened sympathetic nervous system activity. I also learned that taking Valium in bottles at a time didn't help my sex life. Nor much else in my life.

Valium is a benzodiazepine, touted as a tranquilizer that calms without sedating, and less dangerous than the barbiturates it replaced. Barbiturates were a common source of lethal overdoses, and were very sedating. In reality, I found as many others did that Valium is sedating and lethal when taken with any drugs such as opioids and alcohol. Pharmaceutical companies are good at conning doctors, and doctors are easy to con. And if it's addicting, patients want it. I know I did. The problem is that Valium doesn't help, it harms. I had taken handfuls daily, weekly, monthly. So much, so often, I didn't think of sex. Didn't think of much.

Of course, one drug led to another drug, and I was concocting my own cures. I took Valium to ward off the shakes from alcohol, narcotics to substitute for alcohol during the day so I could work, chloral hydrate and later placidly, to sedate arousal from opioids, which I took to anesthetize, numb, and become unconscious. I don't know why I didn't die from my treatment plan. It was particularly harrowing when I drank alcohol. Just how I lived to tell this story, I don't know. Not good at dying, I guess.

You can imagine Johns Hopkins did not recruit me to practice my drug addiction as I did. I continued to take increasingly large amounts of Darvon, Valium, interspersed with Quaaludes. I was a walking pharmacy. My physical condition reflected my choices of drugs. I lost 50 pounds or more, existed on a diet of yogurt to avoid constipation, and developed obsessive-compulsive disorder from perpetual, narcotic intoxication. I was not drinking much alcohol, and actually went a year without it on my substitute narcotics and sedatives, analogous to Hopkins' founder, William Stewart Halstead, and his infamous exchange of morphine for cocaine. That meant I could avoid runs of days and nights that merged when I drank, and not make a spectacular ass of myself at the Department of Psychiatry Journal Club. At Journal Club, grape wine was served, and I poured mine out in intoxicating quantities. What I didn't figure, was just how intoxicated I became when I mixed the wine with the pills I took regularly. I went off into blind rages at the Journal Club. A surprise to all, I imagine.

Early in the beginning of my residency at Hopkins, the Department knew I had a drinking problem. During my residency with them, I had been admitted to three psychiatric hospitals for alcohol intoxication, depression, suicidal behavior, and withdrawal. That period was particularly difficult, as I went from a resident in a psychiatric to a patient in another psychiatric hospital. Learning from both angles, applying my residency experience poorly to my patient experience. You can imagine what great training I was getting, certainly hands on, both as patient and doctor.

By this time, the Department was trying all kinds of treatments to help me. They did not throw me under the bus. The Chair of Psychiatry, Dr. Jack Murphy, had a reputation for loyalty to his followers, as did some of his other faculty. In no way did they judge me, and went out of their way to support me. But they did not understand alcoholism and drug addiction. Did not consider it a disease, rather just a behavior. Since I was still trying to hold on to what I had left of my residency, I had difficulty following their recommendations because I kept drinking and drugging.

Believe it or not, I did learn psychiatry. Dr. Murphy and his staff were brilliant teachers, stressing principles of mental illness, relying on European psychiatrists, British and German. Observation and objectivity were stressed over theory and intuition. Dr. Murphy emphasized what we knew, less than than what we didn't know about mental illness. I can't say that he was right about everything, but I did like his objective, here and now approach, rather than guessing and surmising why people acted and felt as they did.

His psychiatric approach coincided with the movement in the U.S. to diagnose major mental illness, such as manic-depressive illness. Later that nomenclature changed to Bipolar Disorder, stressing the opposite, extreme poles of mood disorders. Mania was elevated mood, hyperactive behaviors, grandiose delusions, hedonistic and hypersexuality, intrusive interpersonal transgressions. At the other extreme pole, was depressed mood, psychomotor retardation or slowed behaviors, self-blame, lack of pleasure, low sexual interests, and poor interpersonal interactions. Manic-Depressive Illness is a remitting and relapsing disorder that often responds well to treatment.

Schizophrenia however, according to Dr. Murphy was over diagnosed, a progressive mental illness, termed "Dementia Precox" or dementing illness in the young due to its devastating, deteriorating effects on personality. Unlike Bipolar Disorder, Schizophrenia was a disorder of thought and perception, with delusions and hallucinations, and did not respond as well to treatment. Dr. Murphy thought everyone then should be considered for Manic Depressive Illness before consigning them to the diagnosis of Schizophrenia with the poorer prognosis.

At first I thought I had schizophrenia, the way I acted and felt. I certainly had a mood disorder with my depression and manic behaviors. However, I did not have either diagnosis, rather I had a progressive, fatal diagnosis of alcohol and drug addiction. I had showed many symptoms of depression, distorted, nearly delusional thinking, aberrant perceptions, and manic hyperactivity. However, on each of my three psychiatric admissions while a resident at Hopkins, I was diagnosed with Alcoholism, and maybe Drug Addiction. I was offered no treatment for alcoholism but was probably referred to AA. I was not given another psychiatric diagnosis, not even antisocial personality disorder. This wouldn't happen today. I certainly would carry the label of bipolar disorder or personality disorder or something psychiatric.

However, drugs or substances including alcohol, induce or cause symptoms of mental illness, not mental illness itself, per say. DSM-5 has exclusionary criteria that require excluding the effects of alcohol and drugs in inducing psychiatric symptoms before making an independent psychiatric diagnosis. Not that many who diagnose respect that rule. The DSM-5 actually has Substance Induced Disorders for the major psychiatric symptoms. Substance Induced Depression and Anxiety are very common in regular use of addicting drugs, medications and alcohol.

While someone is taking these chemicals, it is not possible to make other psychiatric diagnoses until the effects of alcohol and drugs inducing depression, anxiety, hallucinations, and delusions are accounted for. Alcohol is a depressant, as are opioid drugs. Why people continue to use alcohol and so-called painkillers despite depression is due to addiction. Compulsive use of a drug causing depression is ordinarily addiction. In other words, addiction is why someone can't stop using a drug, despite its inducing depression. I became suicidal on alcohol and opioid drugs, but I kept using them. I certainly wasn't enjoying them, but used them anyway. Addiction is the only explanation after awhile.

Same goes for anxiety induced by alcohol and opioids. Most people develop a degree of physical dependence on alcohol and opioid medications. No one can maintain a constant blood level of a drug, so everyone experiences some degree of withdrawal. And the main symptoms of drug withdrawal are anxiety and agitation. Also, drugs irritate the brain chemically so the brain response is irritability and agitation. The brain becomes unbalanced in trying to accommodate the drug effects by reaching a new homeostasis to the presence of the drugs. As soon as the drug effects diminish or begin to wear off, the brain responds with anxiety.

Of course, you can imagine how depressed and anxious an addict becomes when conflicts develop in interpersonal relationships, and medical, legal, psychological adverse consequences ensue. Situational anxiety and depression can be severe and incapacitating. How many times have you been stymied by fear and apprehension? And paralyzed by your feelings?

The centers in the brain for mood regulation contain pathways for addictions. Mood and addiction occur in the limbic lobe in the brain, an area responsible for the instincts as well. Which is why emotions, addiction, and mental disorders are tied to each other, and promote each other. The amygdala in the limbic lobe is part of the brain responsible for aggression and emotions. The mesolimbic pathway consists of dopamine neurons in the brainstem, which synapse or connect with the nucleus accumbens in the limbic lobe to establish an addictive drive to use alcohol and drugs. Emotions, addiction, and sex are closely associated in the limbic system, dating back to early evolution.

The limbic system is one of the oldest parts of the brain because it is responsible for instincts that promote survival, sex, eating, and fight or flight responses. Limbic system sounds like fun, right? Only if under control. An out of control limbic system runs counter to survival and well-being. You can imagine what it would be like if you over ate, had sex all day and night, fought everyone, and ran from yourself.

We treat anxiety and depression as a result of drugs, by abstaining from the offending drugs. Antidepressants and anti-anxiety agents do nothing for drug induced depression and anxiety, and are dangerous to mix. Not to mention, anti-anxiety drugs such as benzodiazepines, Xanax, Valium, Klonopin, are highly addicting, adding another dimension to the problem. Psychotherapy does little to stem the tide of addiction if focused on underlying causes of addictive drug use.

Understanding why someone uses, is fruitless unless aimed at the brain initiated addictive drive. Going back through childhood for answers does not lead to explanations for addictive drug use. Even life's traumas and abuses may trigger drug use, but compulsive use, which develops as a life of its own, is not related to deep underlying psychological problems or a series of bad breaks. Psychotherapy can help if focused on addiction and its specific treatments.

We tried most of these treatment methods except medications, maybe because I was on so many medications the time. Nobody uttered the words alcoholic, alcoholism, drug addiction, drug addict. Nor did I. Those were diagnoses reserved for patients, who usually had personality disorders. Personality disorder people maladapt to life, do bad things to themselves and others, and drink and drug. So I was treated as a characterological defective or inadequate person. I harmed myself and others because I was raised wrong or my personality developed poorly. I reacted to life in ways that were morally offensive, and socially corrupt. I did not have a disease or disorder that could be diagnosed. Rather I had deep rooted psychological problems that caused out of control drinking and drugging. If I could uncover these distorted and twisted attitudes and reactions to life, I would want to be and act normal.

Sigmund Freud was another drug addict. He was addicted to cocaine. Like me, he was a neurologist who became a psychiatrist, though I became a psychiatrist before I became a neurologist. He started with an interest in the brain, and actually studied neuropathology. He developed some of the original microscopic stains for nerve cells. Eventually, he developed an interest in hysteria. Neurologists saw hysteria quite often as it often mimicked neurological symptoms. Freud saw hysterical paralysis as a symptom of psychological trauma.

He treated a patient, Anna O., who had paralysis of extremities, hallucinations, loss of consciousness, and other symptoms. According to hysteria, these symptoms were psychological in origin and nature. Anna did not really have neurological paralysis or altered consciousness; rather, she had developed an abnormal psychological coping with trauma of her father's suffering before his death. She developed hysterical symptoms while caring for her father who died of tuberculosis. Freud's theory was that her father's death was an antecedent psychological trauma that led to her hysterical symptoms. A colleague of Freud, Josef Breuer, used hypnosis to uncover the unconscious antecedent traumatic psychological events. From Breuer's work, Freud developed his theories of the unconscious as he saw hysteria as an abnormal expression of the unconscious experiences.

In Freudian theory, the human mind is structured into

two main parts: the conscious and unconscious mind. The conscious mind includes all the things we are aware of or can easily bring into consciousness. The unconscious mind, on the other hand, includes all of the things outside of our awareness—all of the wishes, desires, hopes, urges, and memories that lie outside of consciousness yet continue to influence our awareness and conscious behavior. Freud compared the mind to an iceberg. The tip of the iceberg that is actually visible above the water represents just a tiny portion of the our mental experiences, while the huge expanse of ice hidden underneath the water represents the much larger unconscious drives and experiences.

In addition to these two main components of the mind, Freudian theory also divides human personality up into three major components: the id, ego and superego. The id is the most primitive part of personality that is the source of all our most basic urges. This part of personality is entirely unconscious and serves as the source of all libidinal energy. The ego is the component of personality that is charged with dealing with reality and helps ensure that the demands of the id are satisfied in ways that are realistic, safe and socially acceptable. The superego is the part of personality that holds all of the internalized morals and standards that we acquire from our parents, family and society at large.

Even if you've never studied Freud's theories before, you have probably heard the term "defense mechanisms" bandied about a few times. When someone seems unwilling to face a painful truth, you might accuse them of being "in denial." When a person tries to look for a logical explanation for unacceptable behavior, you might suggest that they are "rationalizing."

Rationalizations and minimization represent different types of defense mechanisms, or tactics that the ego uses to protect itself from anxiety arising from unconscious conflicts. Some of the best-known mechanisms of defense include denial, repression, and regression, but there are many more. Defense mechanisms are thought to safeguard against feelings and thoughts that are too difficult for the conscious mind to cope with. In some instances, defense mechanisms are thought to keep inappropriate or un-wanted thoughts and impulses from entering the conscious mind.

Because addiction provokes the appetitive drives in the id, and guilt in the superego, the ego employs a number of defense mechanisms to cope with disrupted and disturbed reality caused by addictions. Although we may knowingly use these mechanisms, in many cases these de-fenses work unconsciously to distort our reality to keep us from honestly knowing the nature and consequences from our addictions. My ego was hypertrophied from being over-worked by alcohol and drugs increasing hedonic id impulses and punitive, superego admonishments.

For example, if faced with a particularly unpleasant task, the mind may choose to forget responsibility in order to avoid the dreaded consequences. In addition to forget-ting, other defense mechanisms of rationalization, denial, repression, projection, rejection, and reaction formation thwart unacceptable, painful feelings and experience. I my-self, was a master at forgetting. I just didn't think about my alcohol and drug use, and I carried around a blank slate about its consequences. Being held in jail for drunk driving was just another thing I had to endure, but I had little to do with it. And I certainly did not deal with cause, alcohol.

While all defense mechanisms can be unhealthy, they can also help us adapt and allow us to function normally. Great problems arise when defense mechanisms are overused in order to avoid dealing with problems, such as addiction. In psychoanalytic therapy, the goal may be to help the client uncover these unconscious defense mechanisms and find better, healthier ways of coping with addiction and distress.

Among the several defense mechanisms, denial is the first and foremost mental twist to propagate and sustain addictive use of alcohol and drugs. Denial is probably one of the best known defense mechanisms, used often to describe situations in which people seem unable to face reality or admit an obvious truth (i.e. "He's in denial.") Denial is an outright refusal to admit or recognize that something has occurred or is currently occurring. As I did, drug addicts and alcoholics often deny that they have a problem, while victims of traumatic events may deny that the event ever occurred.

Denial functions to protect the ego from things that the individual cannot cope with. While this may save us from anxiety or pain, denial also requires a substantial investment of energy. Because of this, other defenses are also used to keep these unacceptable feelings from consciousness. In many cases, there might be overwhelming evidence that something is true, yet the person will continue to deny its existence or truth because it is too uncomfortable to face. Does denial make sense?

Denial can involve a complete rejection of the existence of a fact or reality. In other cases, it might involve admitting that something is true, but minimizing its importance. Sometimes people will accept reality and the seriousness of the fact, but they will deny their own responsibility and instead blame other people or other outside forces. I was again a master at admitting I had a problem, but minimized how alcohol and drugs affected my life, and their consequences. I certainly either didn't accept responsibility or cared about how my life was under the control of alcohol and drugs.

Addiction is one of the best-known examples of denial. People who are suffering from addiction problems will often flat-out deny that their behavior is problematic. In other cases, they might admit that they do use drugs or alcohol, but will claim that this addiction was not a problem. That was me. My denial was so great I didn't even think about it. I denied I used alcohol and drugs to myself and others, and denied all the awful things I did to myself and others. I was so good at denial I didn't know why I used, or what it did to me. Denial is lethal.

Repression is another well-known defense mechanism. Repression acts to keep unconscious information out of conscious awareness. However, these memories don't just disappear; they continue to influence our behavior unconsciously. For example, a person who has repressed memories of experiences suffered as a practicing addict may continue to use alcohol and drugs. Sometimes I forced unwanted information out of my awareness, which is known as suppression. In most cases, I just forgot or didn't think at all, mostly didn't think. Problematic addictive drive occurs unconsciously, and I felt like a puppet being controlled and compelled to drink and drug. I just didn't think about what the next drink or drug would do to me, nor did I care.

Projection is a defense mechanism that involves taking our own unacceptable qualities or feelings and ascribing or projecting them to other people. In my case, I would blame others or circumstances for the bad acts caused by drinking, thereby, not facing the realities of my use. Projection worked by allowing the expression of the desire or impulse of my drinking behavior, in a way that the ego or consciousness could not recognize, therefore compounding my addictive use. The world is just a bad place, so naturally, I was not at fault or responsible. I became jaded and cynical with my perceptions of realities and others. It was my mother's fault that I drank. I became the ultimate victim. Did I feel sorry for me? You bet.

Intellectualization worked to reduce anxiety by thinking about events in a cold, clinical way. This defense mechanism allowed me to avoid thinking about the stressful, emotional aspect of my drinking and drug use and instead focus only on the intellectual component. I would describe events to wall off the emotional impact or realities, so as not to experience the consequences of my bad acts when drinking. I was a doctor so I could handle my drinking. I was progressing in my professional life so I couldn't be that bad of an alcoholic. So I thought. I didn't have it figured out and I always thought the next guy was wrong. I had plenty of stories to explain your faults.

Rationalization involves explaining an unacceptable behavior or feeling in a rational or logical manner, avoiding the true reasons for the behavior. Many alcoholics and addicts rationalize or blame their drinking on stress, or other people, childhood, events rather than on themselves. I certainly held many more people accountable for my actions than myself. I had chosen the wrong residency program, or specialty. I lived in the wrong place, that a series of misunderstandings and bad breaks caused my drinking. I was never the problem, someone else was the problem. If you felt ugly and dumb, and looked awful and did dumb things, you wouldn't blame yourself, would you?

Rationalization not only prevented my accurate perception of reality, it also perversely protected my self-esteem and self-concept. When confronted by success or failure, I attributed achievement to my own qualities and skills, while failures were blamed on other people or outside forces. I was always struggling with my self-assessment of my intelligence, doubted it, compared myself to others, and came up short. I felt less or more than, never accurate in my own self-image. I often failed to achieve because of my drinking, but was not able to see how my drinking was the cause. I attributed my failures to me or others, and not my drinking or drug use. I would blame you, if I had the chance.

Reaction formation sustained my addiction as I adopted the opposite feeling, impulse or behavior. I was the doctor, and not the patient. My drinking was not as bad as a patient. According to Freud, I used reaction formation as a defense mechanism to hide my true feelings by behaving in the exact opposite manner. I was acting to treat someone else with the problem so I was not as bad or my drinking was not as bad. Truthfully I just didn't think much, I was living a life of excuses, denial, minimization, projecting my problems with drinking onto others and irrelevant reality. I was living for the next pill, or bottle of pills. Have you ever compared yourself to someone to justify your actions? I did it all the time.

I was not preoccupied with suicidal thoughts consciously. I did not think about how and when I would kill myself. Even when I stocked piled bottles of sedatives, particularly, Quaaludes, powerful respiratory depressants. It was the one pill I did not have to take a lot of to get high or sedated. It was a pill I did not use regularly. My desire to die was as unconscious as my desire to use drugs and alcohol. I was a walking time bomb and didn't know it. What would you do if you had to take so many pills? And didn't know why you were taking them?

I had stopped drinking alcohol completely as I progressively used heavier and more frequent doses of highly addicting sedatives. I could not predict my actions at all. I did not want to end up in jail or hospital where drinking often took me. I replaced my alcohol intoxication with pills, bottles. I spent time making my rounds of pharmacies to prescribe myself the pills, making out the prescriptions to me, my wife, others. I had developed a network of pharmacies to try to stay under the radar. I would write a prescription for Darvon to dispense 100 to 200 capsules at a time. I would probably take 20 to 40 capsules per day in handfuls. I can't tell you just what went through my mind if anything as to when, how many, and why I took the Darvon. Clearly the drug controlled my use as I had to balance withdrawal with intoxication, and nausea, anxiety and insomnia from the Darvon.

I sedated myself with Valium, and later Quaaludes to sleep and come down from the excitement caused by Darvon. I substituted pills for alcohol. It made sense to me at the time. I wouldn't drive in an alcohol blackout, wouldn't be arrested for drunk driving, say stupid things without knowing what I said as I would with alcohol. Do you agree I made a good decision, to substitute one drug for another? Some doctors would say so, they call it medication assisted treatment. A transfer of one drug addiction for another. A popular form of treatment these days. Does that make sense? It didn't ultimately for me.

I lost 50 lbs. or more, weighed 140 lbs. at 6 feet, ½ inch frame. I regularly, manually evacuated my stool because of severe constipation from the opioid drug. I ate very little, mostly just yogurt. I looked funny to people, but then again I was a psychiatrist. I don't think I had much of a sex life at that point, and I slept in a separate bedroom from my wife. I don't recall having many thoughts about much. I just recall emptying bottles of pills, swallowing handfuls of pills, not really counting, not really caring. Meanwhile, I was trying to find out why I took so many pills when I didn't have a physical pain. I think you would agree that I looked sick, felt sick, but wasn't sick except for the pills.

I had started seeing a psychoanalyst for my alcoholism. A nice man, who just let me talk while he was listening. I did not give him any indication of what I was preparing to do nor did I give myself any idea I would try to take my life. Somehow, his theory was simply that I would rid myself of deep rooted psychological causes of my addictions by talking enough for unconscious conflicts to rise to consciousness and eventual resolutions. According to psycholanalytic theory, my earlier experiences dating back to childhood drove me to drink. By "free association" I could rid myself of conflicts that triggered and sustained my addictive drive for alcohol and drug use. A nice theory, and a deadly one.

Psychiatrist Dr. Aaron T. Beck explored the relation of hopelessness to levels of depression and suicidal intent both psychologically and clinically. The results of an investigation of 384 suicide attempters supported previous reports that hopelessness is the key variable linking depression to suicidal behavior. This finding has direct implications for the interventions and therapy of suicidal individuals. By focusing on reducing the sources of a patient's hopelessness, the professional may be able to alleviate suicidal crises more effectively than in the past. However, I couldn't honestly say I felt hopeless. I certainly didn't express it to others; I was determined to advance my career one pill at a time.

He also did a prospective study of 1,958 outpatients

and found that hopelessness, as measured by the Beck Hopelessness Scale, was significantly related to eventual suicide. A scale cutoff score of 9 or above identified 16 (94.2%) of the 17 patients who eventually committed suicide, thus replicating a previous study with hospitalized patients. The high-risk group identified by this cutoff score was 11 times more likely to commit suicide than the rest of the outpatients. I felt hopeless but did not know it.

The Substance Abuse and Mental Health Services Administration (SAMHSA) states that suicide kills more than 39,000 people a year in the United States. That's an average of 108 suicides each day. Additional data from the Centers for Disease Control (CDC) reveals suicide is the 10th leading cause of death in the United States, with alcohol and drug addicts being six times more likely to take their own lives. While depression and other mood disorders are the number-one risk factor for suicide, alcohol and drug addiction (even without the diagnosis of depression), are ranked a close second. In fact, other research has shown that the strongest predictor of suicide is not a psychiatric diagnosis —but alcoholism and drug addiction. I didn't predict suicide for myself but it almost happened.

You wonder why I used drugs when they are so dangerous. I did too. You can call me stupid. I sure acted like it. Addiction not only increases the likelihood a person will take his or her own life, the disease itself is used as a method of committing suicide, drug by drug. According to data from the National Alliance on Mental Illness, one in three people who die from suicide are under the influence of drugs—typically opiates (oxycodone or heroin) or alcohol. Poisoning is the third-leading method used in suicide deaths and drugs make up 75% of suicide deaths caused by poisoning. I had several bouts with suicide, and up to now I had won. You decide if surviving or dying is winning or losing, if addicted to drugs.

Johns Hopkins Hospital earned its reputation that day as they performed a procedure only tried six times previously in the world. The day the doctors flushed dialyzed charcoal through my blood (to absorb the drugs before they could completely suppress my respirations, blood pressure and pulse, and turn my brain to jelly), I was placed on a ventilator. I remained in a coma, unresponsive, for four days. I woke in the recovery room to a nurse and resident doctor who tried to explain I had just tried to kill myself. Well, I already knew that. What I didn't know was, why? Not for a moment.

My denial ultimately failed me. My first conscious thought was disappointment. I could neither live nor kill myself. An utmost failure. Though I had no prior thoughts of killing myself, I knew what I had tried to do when I woke up. I was not thrilled to be alive. I was still full of anger and self-hate, that sense of failure. Then suddenly, the miracle happened. I finally realized I had escaped death. And I wrote on a clip board the nurse had given me, "Hope Springs Eternal," Just why I knew not, but the thought came none too soon.

Hope springs eternal in the human breast;
Man never is, but always to be blessed:
The soul, uneasy and confined from home,
Rests and expatiates in a life to come.

—"An Essay on Man" Alexander Pope

PART II.
WHAT HAPPENED

8

POWERLESSNESS AND ACCEPTANCE

"Ruin and recovery are both from within."
—Epicterus

"Who cares to admit complete defeat? Practically no one, of course. Every natural instinct cries out against the idea of personal powerlessness. It is truly awful to admit that, glass in hand, we have warped our minds into such an obsession for destructive drinking that only an act of Providence can remove it from us." —Twelve Steps and Twelve Traditions, Alcoholics Anonymous World Services, Inc.

Next, I found myself in a Cardiac Intensive Care Unit, wired up to monitors, glaring lights staring me in face, an overwhelming stimulation, with plain, white background. No wonder patients become delirious in ICUs. I suppose I was being monitored because of possible cardiac arrhythmias from Darvon. I don't recall being given medications for withdrawal from sedatives, opioids, and other drugs. Man's Best Doctors could save my life but could not treat drug withdrawal. In drug withdrawal, I felt wired, like I was going to burst. That was tough work for me, beginning to see what it would be like to save my life, rather than ending it. I remember doctors coming in to talk with me. Not much happened. I don't think I slept. After a few days of observation, and no cardiac events, I was placed in a wheelchair and hauled out of Man's Best Hospital unceremoniously. I could barely stand, weighed a mere smidgen of my former self. I certainly didn't feel like a hero. Still not dedicated to living, still believing I could do it all on my own.

Next, I found myself in yet another psychiatric hospital. Somehow they had deduced I had attempted suicide, I guess. I bet you are not surprised to find this out. Just how many of you feel sorry for me? I of course, did it all to myself, so why should anyone pity me? But I did. Self-will run riot, and I was in the driver's seat, racing aimlessly towards self-destruction. I was helpless in the face of a mental obsession and compulsion to drink. No matter what the consequences, even if I had entertained them, which I often didn't, I picked up the next drink in a determined drive to oblivion.

To this day, I do not know or understand why I chose misery and suffering, but I did, over and over again, without fail. The mental obsession with alcohol was beyond my willpower, and any resistance I attempted against the first drink, was often too little. Once the first drink was taken, the compulsion set in, and I was overtaken by the drive to the next drink, after drink, to oblivion. My aim was unconscious blackout. My motto was, "There will be no stopping." I didn't choose my next drink; it chose me, over and over again.

Whatever I did with alcohol, I did the same with pills. Darvon, Valium, Quaaludes had the same effects on me as alcohol. What I didn't realize at the time was I could not solve my problems with the same thinking I used when I created them. With pills I was more conscious, had fewer blackouts, and until my unconscious overdose, had avoided hospitals and jails. I was just as powerless over drugs as alcohol, and my life had become equally unmanageable. I could not break my preoccupation with intoxicating oblivion and lowly self-hatred. I was on a merry-go-round without

merriment. Without memory, I can say I lived with determination to forget, to fail, to avoid fear, and to humiliate
myself. I kept going lower and lower, and never seeming to
reach a bottom. Where would it end?

I instinctively did not think sitting in a psychiatric
ward was the answer. I couldn't see solutions in making
moccasins, and listening to the usual explanations that did
not make sense or, more importantly, work for me.

Therapist A told me I suffered from a self-inflicted
moral problem, and that I just needed to get right with myself and understand what I was doing to myself. That I do
not need medical or psychological treatment, I just simply
needed to pull myself up by my boot straps and exert my
willpower to control my drinking. Either by myself or just
staying away from it.

Therapist B told me I suffered from a personality or
character disorder and needed long-term psychoanalysis to
understand how my job and early childhood influenced my
reactions to life. I was encouraged to change my personality by digging deeply into my unconscious mind, (below the
surface of what I can remember), to understand my basic
motivations. Ultimately, I would be able to take alcohol and
other psychoactive drugs, because the underlying problems
would no longer cause me the psychic pain I supposedly relieved with alcohol and drugs.

Therapist C told me that I suffered from an underlying anxiety and depression that caused me to drink or use
drugs, and that I needed antidepressant and anti-anxiety
medications. Also, that I needed psychotherapy to understand why I drank, and what feelings I was trying to cover
up or relieve with alcohol and drugs. Once my anxiety and
depression were treated, I will either not need to drink, or
be able to moderate my drinking because my mood would

no longer need if medicating.

Therapist D told me I had low self-esteem, lacked social skills, and needed psychological help to learn how to relate better to people. If I corrected these deficits, I could control my drinking and drug use by staying away from people, places, and things that I associated with alcohol and drugs.

So I did what I always did, and that was to sign out AMA or against medical advice. My wife signed the release even after finding me nearly dead just two weeks prior. But the next thing I did was return to my shrink, the psychoanalyst who was trying to illicit why I drank and did the crazy things I did. Guess what he did? He asked, first thing, if I had been treated with Lithium in the psychiatric hospital, and I said no. Next, he offered me the name of a physician who he said would take me to a meeting of Alcoholics Anonymous. He said the doctor would call me. Sure enough he did call, and I agreed to go. What I haven't told you yet is that I started to drink alcohol shortly after arriving home from the ICU and funny farm. I was off to the races, and was drinking where I had left off, in bottles. But I had not taken any pills yet. I probably associated pills with death.

My future AA sponsor arrived at my townhouse. He was a short, pleasant, gentlemanly man who liked to talk, not giving me a chance to interrupt with my objections, excuses, and belligerent distractions. He immediately said, "You need to go into a treatment center, I have never seen anyone as sick as you. I have never seen anyone take as many drugs, and you look terrible." He had a professional basis for that opinion, as he was a Johns Hopkins trained surgeon, who practiced surgery in the area. He also had years of recovery in AA, and was full of AA sayings, exhortations, and a funny laugh with his numerous comments.

He took me to me to a physicians' AA meeting, a rather large group of doctors. I heard I had the disease of alcoholism. I was told I have a *disease*, like diabetes, hypertension, cancer. And that I needed treatment. That treatment was AA. But the most important instruction I gleaned that day, as I tried to stand, reeking with alcohol from the night before, came unexpectedly. A robust, large man with a bald head, leaned over and said, "You are insane." I didn't flinch. I instinctively knew what he was saying. I deduced, I had to be insane to be in a room of alcoholic doctors to begin with. And I had just been released from an intensive care unit after a fatal overdose only Man's Best Hospital could reincarnate, signed out against medical advice from a psychiatric hospital after a nearly completed suicide, and started to drink again, and I mean drink. Bottles of whiskey and wine, right where I left off.

My self-appointed AA sponsor told me that I suffer from a physical, mental, and spiritual disease, and needed 12 Step treatment to stop drinking and using drugs. This 12 Step treatment will have physical, psychological, and spiritual elements to its ingredients. I am told I am anxious and depressed, and I need to abstain from alcohol and other drugs to feel better, and to go on to change my thinking and feelings.

My sponsor told me that insanity is doing the same thing over and over again, and expecting different results. He must have read Einstein, who had said that too. Every time I picked up a drink or pill, I experienced the same consequences. That is addiction. I heard at AA meetings that I had to change my thinking, and could not expect to solve my problems with the same thinking I used to create the problems. Can you believe these were novel ideas? I had to acknowledge I was insane to change.

Hearing I had a disease was very helpful to begin to assuage the guilt and self-loathing I had created in my addictive use of drugs and alcohol. That I was not at fault for my addictive disease, relieved me of suicidal thinking. But I was not left off the hook, as I am responsible for my recovery from addictive disease. Just like someone with diabetes or hypertension, they are not at fault for the disease, but are responsible for taking insulin or antihypertensive medications to treat their conditions.

But you say the alcoholic or drug addict started using in the first place. So you say they are at fault. Then I say, if gaining weight causes some forms of diabetes and hypertension is that not the same thing as initiating drinking or drug use? Guess what? How many people with diabetes and hypertension take their medications as directed? About only one quarter of these patients comply with directions for taking these medications. Yet we don't tag them with a moral problem as we do alcoholics who don't seek or accept treatment. Even cancer, which is out of control growth of cells, can have origins in behavior, e.g. smoking cigarettes for lung cancer, having sexually transmitted disease in cervical cancer, or poor diet in colon cancer. Do you consider them sinners if they don't take steps to prevent their cancers? We just maybe say they should have exercised better judgment or made better decisions. But you don't hold them at fault; after all they have a disease.

You might be surprised that courts view alcoholism and drug addiction as diseases. The California Supreme Court held that drug addiction is a status, not a crime, when it ruled that the California law making drug addiction a crime was unconstitutional. Moreover, the Court distinguished treatment and punishment as two different goals in drug addiction. Similarly, the U.S. Supreme Court ruled that public drunkenness was a crime but that being an alcoholic was not a crime. A Maryland Court ruling illustrates the legal approach to alcoholism (drug addiction) as a disease. The court ruled:

> There is no evidence on the record legally sufficient for the jury to find the chronic alcoholism of the insured is a result of his conscious purpose or design. On the contrary, that testimony tends to show that he had vainly exercised his will to restrain a control his desire. The result of his disease is a weakness of the will and character, which caused him to yield the liquors. The drinking in the first stages was voluntary but there was not testimony that the drinker was aware of the latent danger in his habit: and so while his consumption of liquor was a voluntary act, yet his ignorance of its insidious effect does not make the act voluntary exposure of himself to the unapprehended and unexpected danger of the disease of chronic alcoholism. The result of the indulgence of an appetite does not necessarily determine that the result was self-inflicted because the actor does not apprehend or is ignorant of the danger of his act.

Courts on the local level, particularly, trial courts allow for the involuntary nature of alcohol/drug addiction. Generally, they will mitigate the legal consequences in charges and sentencing, and accept as a retribution the rehabilitation treatment and commitment to recovery by the offender. As many as one third of those who enter and become members of Alcoholics Anonymous are referred by the courts. Actually, coerced treatment mandated by the courts is more effective than voluntary treatment because those coerced generally enter treatment at an earlier course in their addictive disease. Whereas those who wait until "they are ready" accrued greater consequences and are sicker and more affected by their addictive diseases.

Are you one of those who think addiction is due to a moral problem or sin or evil? Most of us do, to some extent. I especially felt guilt laden with sin during my drinking and drug days. In some ways a moral view encourages continued drug use because of the guilt caused by consequences. The addict may look defiant on the outside, but inside their self-condemnation is deep and painful. They hate themselves, and therefore, the world outside. Religious attempts to purge the sinner from curse of addiction are sometimes successful but often fall short of accepting the core biological and mental causes of addiction.

Despite the prevalent moral view, I have yet to find a medical study that links immorality with addictive drug and alcohol use. Morality makes the most sense if you apply it to goodness or rightness in addiction. You can understand that harming oneself and others is not good or right. But immorality is a common consequence of addictive use of alcohol and drugs, and not the cause of it. We do not do good things or act right because we are compelled by our addictive use. We often fail in being good and acting right but don't become alcoholics or addicts.

Actually, the frontal lobe in the brain is responsible for ethical or proper behaviors. Alcohol and drugs impair or suppress frontal lobe activity so we act improper or unethical when alcohol and drugs drench our frontal lobes. Demented people who suffer from degeneration of their frontal lobes will show improper behaviors with sexuality, toilet functions, etc., functions which come under the control of the frontal lobe under normal conditions.

Another common view is that addiction is the result of a personality or character disorder, and requires long-term psychoanalysis to understand how early childhood influences reactions to life. I am encouraged to change my personality by digging deeply into my unconscious mind (below the surface of what I can remember) and to understand my basic motivations. Ultimately, I will be able to take alcohol and other psychoactive drugs safely, because the underlying problems will no longer cause me the psychic pain I supposedly relieved using alcohol and drugs.

Personality, defined psychologically, is the set of enduring behavioral and mental traits that distinguish humans. Hence, personality disorders are defined by experiences and behaviors that differ from societal norms and expectations. Those diagnosed with a personality disorder may experience difficulties in cognition, emotiveness, interpersonal functioning, or impulse control. In general, personality disorders are diagnosed in 40–60% of psychiatric patients, making them the most frequent of all psychiatric diagnoses.

The DSM-5 provides a definition of a General Personality Disorder that stress such disorders are an enduring and inflexible pattern of long duration that lead to significant distress or impairment and *are not due to use of substances or another medical condition.*

On the other hand, active alcoholics and drug addicts look like they have personality disorders with inflexible personalities, impulsive control, emotional turmoil, maladaptive behaviors, interpersonal difficulties, legal problems, etc. However, these are consequences, and not causes, of out of control alcohol and drug use. Addiction itself is an uncontrolled state of drug use that propels personal conflicts in many spheres of their lives.

What's really remarkable are the personality changes that occur in someone abstinent and in recovery from addiction. The 12 Steps of Alcoholics Anonymous promote change in personality, attitudes, emotions, and interpersonal relationships; promoting fundamental changes in mind, body, and spirit. My personality is certainly more responsible and attentive to the needs of others, whereas in my drugging days I was solely focused on me, myself, and I. At the cost of others.

A very popular, intuitive explanation for addictive use is that I suffered from an underlying anxiety and depression that caused me to drink or use drugs. And that I needed antidepressant and anti-anxiety medications to treat those causes of addictive use, as well as psychotherapy to understand why I drank and what feelings I am trying to cover up or relieve with alcohol and drugs. Once my anxiety and depression were treated, I would either not need to drink, or be able to moderate my drinking because my mood would no longer need self-medicating.

My anxiety and depression worsened with continued alcohol and drug use, to the obvious point I took a near lethal overdose. And the anxiety and depression resolved once I stopped using alcohol and drugs. Addictive use is tricky, as it makes you think drugs are helping when truly they are the problem. Drinkers and drug users often say they use because of anxiety and depression, but actually continue to use despite substance induced mood disturbances.

In one study, a group of patients with manic-depressive illness were followed longitudinally and their drinking actually decreased during depressive episodes, not increased. Only alcoholics continue to drink during the depressive episodes because of their addictive drive and compulsive use, despite increasing depression. Studies and clinical experience show that anxiety and depressive symptoms are increased during alcohol and drug use, and remit with abstinence. Abstinence correlates best with normal mood. Suicide correlates with intoxication, not abstinence.

The self-medication hypothesis proscribes I drank because I had low self-esteem, lacked social skills, and needed psychological help to learn how to relate better to people. If I corrected these psychological deficits, I could control my drinking and drug use by staying away from people, places, and things that I associated with alcohol and drugs. As psychologically appealing as these explanations appeared, I sought alcohol and drugs that led to very low self-esteem. I constantly thought myself to be less than, didn't fit in, different from others, dumb, ugly and doomed, and these feelings worsened with advancing drug and alcohol use. Because I could not predict my psychological state or behaviors while using, I had no confidence, and worried what I would do in my next black out; how I would embarrass myself. I could not look people in the eyes. I shunned the world. I walked in the valley of death, while fearing everyone and everything.

I was constantly trying to explain my irrational thoughts and behaviors. I had intellectualized my entire world. I had rationalizations for just about everything. I lived in complete denial of my addiction and the life it created. I feared shadows, running away from ghosts of the past, present, and future, and my impending doom. When would the next tsunami hit? I was a walking time bomb, sure to go off. On a roller coaster, out of control, heading for a disaster. Death only a matter of time; committed to dying, sure to happen. No way to live. Not living, just along for the ride with death.

One day, I was looking out the window of my townhouse on a dreary afternoon in late October. I thought to myself, if I keep drinking I would be sure to start back using the tranquilizers, sedatives, and narcotics, etc. I would over-dose next, followed by another intensive care unit, psychi-atric hospital, alcohol. *I wasn't afraid of death. I was afraid of living.* I had had enough. I had reached my bottom. I was trapped somewhere between living and dying, in limbo, on the fence, the most difficult place to be. I couldn't stay sober, and couldn't stay drunk. I was a cat on a hot tin roof, unable to stay airborne. I began my long journey of surren-der to win. I had to give up alcohol and drugs for good, one day at a time. I had to acknowledge I was powerless over al-cohol and drugs; imagine, finally.

A feeling came over me, call it divine providence, sane thinking, logical deduction, a moment of clarity, an epiphany or accident, or just plain dumb luck. As I searched the grey day for answers, *I made a decision to live.* Not sur-prisingly, the next thought was I could not ever use alcohol or drugs; they had to leave my life if I expected to live. Thus, my first decision was not to quit using alcohol and drugs. I had made that decision a thousand times. But I had never made a commitment to live. I had arrived at Step 1.

AA Step 1: "We admitted we were powerless over al-cohol- that our lives had become unmanageable." The prin-ciple for this step is acceptance. Next, I had to admit I was powerless over alcohol and drugs and my life had become unmanageable. You may think I was crazy not to know that; you are right, I was insane. But I just couldn't admit I was powerless. Believe it not, I remained tentative about my decision to live. I started attending AA on a day-to-day, trial basis. I liked the day at a time concept. I was not dedicated to living more than a day at a time anyway, as one drink or one drug at a time was intuitive to me. I certainly wasn't sure I wanted to attend AA indefinitely or even stay sober for that matter.

My sponsor started to pick me up for meetings. As I rode in the car with him, he gave me advice on the power greater than myself, "Make believe, if you don't believe." I had such a conflicted religious background, Christ or no Christ, believe or don't believe. I felt deserted and abandoned by my God. I had long forsaken any higher power in my life besides my addiction. I was powerless over alcohol and drugs, so I drank and swallowed pills. I had given up all choice, I was compelled. My dilemma was a *lack of power.*

AA Step 2: "Came to believe that a power greater than myself could restore me to sanity." From the time the big, bald man labeled me, I instinctively knew I was insane. I kept doing the same things, and getting the same, bad results. The principle behind Step 2 is hope. I had long given up hope. Gradually, I began to see in others in AA hope that I could stop using drugs and alcohol. They seemed content without the desperation of the next drink or drug. In fact, they seemed relieved of the God-awful compulsion to drink. I looked up on the wall of a church where I attended AA meetings, and saw a poster of the 12 Steps, and read the second step. I suddenly realized I had hope. It was about two months into my sobriety in AA. What a wonderful feeling, money can't buy, and I couldn't make happen no matter how hard I tried. A gift without a price.

My sponsor and I discussed my returning to my residency training. I had been terminated from Johns Hopkins for drug and alcohol addiction. At the time, I had little desire to return to my Psychiatry residency; I had totally humiliated myself to everyone. Not only had I been treated in the ICU, and exposed my rear-end to the medical world in my gown, I had admitted defeat. I was finally starting to come to terms with my addictions. Because I had been an escape artist, I had already applied for residencies in Neurology prior to my overdose. Dr. Murphy had inspired my interest in Neurology and how it applied to Psychiatry. I had been accepted in several programs. Somehow my sordid, drunken past had not yet caught up with me.

I chose a program in Washington, D.C., Georgetown University Hospital. I started my residency at Georgetown on January 1, 1979, exactly two months after I took my last drink on November 1, 1978, and about three months after I was wheeled out of the ICU. I started to work 90-100 hours per week right off the bat in my Neurology residency. While difficult, due to my protracted withdrawal from drugs, it was still easier sober, than drunk or drugged. I was irritable and hard to deal with, but certainly more reliable.

Needless to say I was pretty shaky, still having muscle twitching from my protracted withdrawal from sedatives, Valium, Quaalude, and opioids, propoxyphene. I felt my raw nerves, and was very moody. I was living about an hour from D.C. so I had a long drive on top of my long hours in the hospital. I was still going to AA meetings. On my first drive to D.C., I had an overwhelming urge to drink. It was so strong I practically lost control of the car. My reflexive reaction was to say to myself, "Let go, let God," and the gripping urge left me. I continued my drive to D.C., and my Neurology residency.

In the meantime, I had applied to and was accepted to a Neurology residency at the University of Minnesota. I can't explain why, but I decided to leave Georgetown, to return to my roots in the Midwest. Maybe I was trying to change people, places, and things, as I did serious damage to myself and others while living in D.C., where I had done very heavy drinking and started my pill use in medical school. And I had done plenty of running from my past with minimal consequences to my ability to move on in places in my career. Little did I know, that my decision to move to Minneapolis/St. Paul was to find Nirvana in my AA recovery. Nirvana is a place and state of perfect quietude, freedom, highest happiness, along with liberation from *samsara*, the repeating cycle of birth, life, and death in my addictions.

*And both that morning equally lay
In leaves no step had trodden black.
Oh, I kept the first for another day!
Yet knowing how way leads on to way
I doubted if I should ever come back.
I shall be telling this with a sigh*

*Somewhere ages and ages hence:
Two roads diverged in a wood, and I,
I took the one less traveled by,
And that has made all the difference.*

—"The Road Not Taken" Robert Frost

9

MADE A DECISION
(Residence, Clinical Pharmacology)

*"Nothing is so exhausting as indecision,
and nothing is so futile."* —Betrand Russell

I almost didn't get a medical license because I lied on the application, not completely on my own, I thought. I had just arrived and I was already in trouble. I answered, "No" to a question asking if I had ever had treatment for a drug or alcohol problem. I swear I followed the suggestion of a prominent physician in the state. I thought he said I didn't have to reveal that information for some reason. Maybe he didn't understand the question but I had later conflicts with him. The Minnesota State Licensing Board found out I had been terminated from my residency at John Hopkins, and wanted to know why I had answered the questions negatively regarding disciplinary actions from problems with drugs and alcohol in the past. I had been sober for about a year, and in recovery in AA. I was supposed to answer that question openly and honestly, they thought. To this day, I felt I did at the time. My twisted, addicted mind took quite some time to think straight, as I spent so many years contriving and lying.

Anyway, I appeared before the entire medical board with my new AA sponsor and the physician who had advised me. I was granted a full medical license by a margin of one vote, with the stipulation I report to a member of the medical board for two years, which I did satisfactorily. However, I got a rude awaking to stigma and prejudice. I was well on my way to correcting my problems, yet the board would barely grant me a medical license, and then required I be monitored. I wonder what their response would be if I answered questions the same way related to medical conditions such as heart disease, diabetes, and even dementia. Probably just a pat on the head, with a request to check in now and then.

I bet you get the idea that I was adept at jumping from one fire to the next, drunk or sober. That could still be true. I certainly lacked judgment, and had a hard time shaking my habit to evade the truth or, more accurately, avoid the consequences from my problems with drugs and alcohol. I was still running a mile a minute, trying to handle it all myself, staying one step ahead of catastrophe, waiting for another explosion; desperately trying to avoid the first drink and drug.

I started to accumulate a number of sayings that I could comprehend and apply to my recovery. "Let go, let God," was a frequent affirmation that seemed to work when impulses or urges to use overwhelmed me. The prerequisite to Step 3 was *willingness*. I certainly knew what willfulness meant in my addiction. I learned in AA meetings that in order for me to stay sober, I had to believe in a power greater than myself. I intuitively knew what that meant as I had turned my will and life over to alcohol and drugs, completely, as I showed little control over their use on my own. Somehow, I had to let go of my attempts to control my use of alcohol and not use drugs, and rely on another power than my own.

I had to learn a new way to stay sober that I did not know or understand. The cardinal manifestation of addiction is the loss of control and poor judgment as a result. At times I was like a bulldozer, trying to overpower, pushing the envelope, crashing into mountains, and meeting up with retaliation. Retaliation became a persistent theme in my life, receiving a blow after I poked someone in the eye. Even when I knew I would be hit, like a boxer, I would continue to swing. I often led with my chin, dropping my gloves, taking full blows. Since my dilemma was a lack of power, I came to Step 3.

Step 3: "Made a decision to turn our will and our lives over to the care of God as we understand Him." Some initially have a hard time with this step, because of conflicting feelings about religion or because they do not believe in God. However, this step isn't meant to be a religious obligation; it's meant to instill addicts with a power to rely on something other than themselves, to help them abstain from drinking alcohol and using drugs. There are several ways recovering alcoholics can use this step to make changes in their lives. Step 3 is like opening a locked door. For me, I wondered, *how shall I let God into my life after He deserted me?*

The Step is clear that at this point, I only needed to "*make a decision,*" and completely turn my life and will over to God. *Willingness* was the key. Dependence on a higher or greater power was a means to independence. I was gradually learning sober the dangers of self-sufficiency and how I experienced the misuse of willpower. What I needed to do was quell the God-awful compulsion of the first drink, and to apply a personal exertion necessary to conform to God's will.

So I made the decision to turn my will over to a

higher power. While I like the word God, I prefer to stay away from a too personal power, especially with religious connotations. I had had my fill of conflicting doctrines, sin and guilt, bossy do's and don'ts. What I needed was power, not religion. In my own mind, Step 3 was the decision to affirm my desire not to drink and use drugs, and establish a commitment to avoid the next drink or drug with the help of a power greater than myself.

I hope you understand that this step, more than any other, in my opinion, ensures the success of the addict, and the program of recovery of Alcoholics Anonymous or Narcotics Anonymous. You see it says the care of God, as *we understood him.* I get to choose my own higher power, not yours or someone else's. Because I had trouble with a human, interventionalist God, I decided on Aristotle's Unmoved Mover as a description of my power.

Aristotle defined his Unmoved Mover as the final and efficient cause. Meaning that it is eternal, and always existed, and will always exist, as a final cause. While it does not move itself, being efficient, it moves everything else, including me. A final cause is the ultimate God, who caused everything, including me, however, humbling that may be. No need to go further into existence. Some refer to it as the first cause, whatever started everything off. I am not sure of the difference; the first cause to me seems to be the final cause. According to Aristotle in *On The Heavens,*

> The unmoved movers, if they were anywhere, were said to fill the outer void, beyond the sphere of fixed stars: It is clear then that there is neither place, nor void, nor time, outside the heaven. Hence whatever is there, is of such a nature as not to occupy any place, nor does time age it; nor is there any change in any of the things which lie beyond the outermost motion; they continue

through their entire duration unalterable and unmodified, living the best and most self- sufficient of lives... From [the fulfillment of the whole heaven] derive the being and life which other things, some more or less articulately but other feebly, enjoy.

It is a power greater than myself that I can approach, seek, and utilize. For me, it is not a divine intervention, it does not seek me out, and only intervenes with its power when I seek or ask for it. Moreover, it is neither male nor female, human nor the man made deity from organized religion. It makes no demands on me, nor do I on it. It is a power I can use to change myself, no one else. I can't make it do anything, but I can use it to make me do anything. I am in control, not it. I derive energy and directions. I call on it to keep me from a drink or drug.

Importantly, it is a perfect mover, yet does not move itself, and I am moved only so perfectly as I seek to be moved by it. It aids my lack of power against the first drink or drug. In the compulsion from addiction, one drink is too many, and a thousand is not enough. I turn my life and my will over to a higher power to quiet my addictive urges, repetitive drive to use, and to change my personality, attitudes, emotions, and perspectives to live more harmoniously with myself and others.

You must be saying at this point, I am making things up, and I could just abstain on my own. However, my experience over the years taught me the contrary, as alone, I am unable to resist the next drink or drug. Sooner or later, the addictive drive will erupt, and I will ignite the compulsive use that will lead me to more and more. You ask, why I would pick up when another drink or drug would make matters worse? I cannot provide a rational answer. Often, I had no thoughts or feelings before the first use, except the quiet before the storm. I did not think the drink through. I did not see the ruin. I was not one to have cravings or pain, or reasons why I drank. I just did and did.

I suppose I convinced myself I drank because I was happy or sad, that I wanted to celebrate, to commiserate, to remember, to forget, for the morning, the night, birthdays, funerals. You name it, that's why I drank. It was mostly for no special reason. As for drugs, I had little prior thoughts, except I had reasoned it helped me to avoid drinking. I actually avoided alcohol for over a year while consuming opioids and sedatives pills. All I was doing was to substitute one substance for another, and while the effects were somewhat different, the results were ultimately the same. I completely forgot that nothing was so bad, that a drink or drug would not make it worse. Now, a higher power gave me time to think, think, think, and think a drink or drug through.

As I attended AA and established a commitment to recovery, my desire to stop drinking and using drugs grew into decisions to commit to abstinence. I made a decision to turn my will and my life over to the care of a power greater than myself or the God of my understanding. You ask, how do I turn my life and will over to the care of God? I answer, one day at a time. I worked the remaining nine steps gradually, really a lifetime to stay away from that first drink and drug.

But I didn't join a monastery, or cult; rather I joined reality, as frightening and ugly as it could be, or as enlightening and beautiful as I wanted it to be. The bottom line being that, in order to refrain from the first addictive use, I had to accept a God or Higher Power to help me. Since it was a power greater than myself, I had to seek it. For I couldn't just wait for the power to invade me, rather I had to pursue it. I got to make my own roadmap, steer my own course, and draw on the power of my unmoved mover. My life in recovery was not all ecclesiastical. I had begun a residency in Neurology at the University of Minnesota, this time sober; a much different atmosphere for me. To begin with, I could show up. I agree with Woody Allen when he said, "Ninety percent of life is showing up." With a brand new feeling, I woke up early in the morning clear headed, with energy and resolve, with direction and promise for completion. I could accumulate information, apply it, and build a store of knowledge and skill. I was encouraged by my mentors with their feedback; I had acquired self-respect, and respect of others, made fewer excuses, was able think with much effort. I was working 90-100 hours per week in my Neurology residency, a grueling and taxing time. I kept close to my AA meetings and friends. I had become a "group project" according to my AA sponsor.

My world was still pretty rough, emotions raw, with a constant headache. From persistent drug effects, I continued to have suicidal thoughts, my muscles drawn tightly, and my mind felt in a vice. I couldn't picture my thoughts, and had little consciousness of myself. I reasoned I was withdrawing from enormous amounts of Valium, Darvon, Quaaludes. Each drug has a prolonged, protracted withdrawal, lasting months to years. I felt at times I would explode. I wished I could have walked in front of a Mack truck, and get it over with.

It took some time, gradually over months, and years for these feelings and sensations to resolve. I didn't take pills nor did I seek physician advice. I spoke to other AA members who had taken similar quantities of these pills, relating similar experiences. Some would laugh and most would tell me to just, "Keep coming back, it gets better."

Because they looked better, and didn't take my torments too seriously, I kept wanting to know how long it would take for me to feel better. Though the sensation of being clean and sober, able to wear fresh and presentable clothes, look the part of a doctor instead of an addict, kept me moving forward.

"Commitment" is the principle behind Step 3. Little did I know that commitment was necessary to stay clean and sober. Studies show that the best predictor of abstinence from alcohol and drugs is the commitment to recovery. I attended many AA meetings. I had moved to St. Paul where a club was located that held many AA meetings going on simultaneously. They were mostly Step meetings, discussing one step per meeting. The groups were relatively small, a dozen or more, breaking up into smaller groups as necessary by counting off.

My wife had followed me to Minnesota, and was a great help in assisting in the transition to the Midwest and sobriety. However, I soon realized that she was not a long-term commitment for me to keep. She was considerably older than I, and I had married her to avoid AA as a solution to my drinking. She was a kind woman, who succeeded in saving my life and ultimately finding AA, ironically. However, I wanted to have children and she probably could not, because of her age. She was a lovely woman who was not the right fit for me in my new, sober life. So I started my sexual liberation, and exploration, this time without intoxicants. I had no idea what sex would be like sober. Another spiritual awakening awaited me.

While I was working as a resident in the hospital, I met a young, beautiful, blonde, Norwegian woman. She was a Computed Tomography (CT) technician who I would converse with, when I read my CT on patients I was caring for. She could actually read the CT scan to help me in the beginning of my residency. Of course, one thing led to another, and I found myself asking her out. I didn't realize she was recently separated from her husband. Before I knew it, I was in her bedroom, looking at her smoothly sculptured body, white and soft. I was worried I couldn't get an erection and sustain a sexual ejaculation. As I discovered I could in fact, perform, I thought to myself, "The program works."

It was such a wonderful experience to know what is was like to feel a woman sober, a first to me. All the other intimate sexual encounters were associated with my drinking and drug use. I really enjoyed exploring her curves and sensuous excitement. We stayed together for a while, but she was hesitant about a committed relationship, I know not why. Maybe she was still tied to her husband or I was just too wild at the time.

I met another young woman in the program who was very sexy and physically gifted. She stayed late after a party one night, and one thing led to another and we ended up together in her bed. By this time, I was feeling better, and could really feel the pleasure from a sexual act. I can still visualize her perfect breasts, and tapered waist. To me she looked like Elizabeth Taylor, sensuous lips to match the rest of her. I was getting adventurous and probably lacked intimate feelings. I wasn't ready to reciprocate to her desire for a commitment beyond sexuality.

I made another change in my relationships when I decided to divorce my wife. While she was a wonderful woman, I had other plans for my life, which would be difficult for her to fill. Our separation and divorce was amiable. Just maybe she had had enough of my harrowing life as a drug addict and alcoholic, and did not want to find me dead someday. I called on my friend who gave me the wedding present of a free divorce. He dispatched my marriage in short order, a marriage dissolved in alcohol and drugs. I have not seen her since.

I met the next woman while I was a resident neurologist serving a rotation in the student health center. She was passionate, aspiring actress, gorgeous, and with whom I had exciting and frequent passionate love making, mixed with spirited, angry arguments, and friction over who knew what. It was all volatility and passion. She seemed interested in my alcoholic background. As I did a physical examination on her, she kind of gave me the eye, and I did the same to her.

I somehow got her telephone number, and called her later. Since she did not continue as a patient with me, I felt I could call her for a personal follow-up. She was seeing someone at the time, but asked me to wait until she could end the relationship. I decided I sure could wait for a beautiful woman! She was strikingly attractive, and was allured by my commitment to AA. She attended open meetings with me.

We had a tumultuous relationship, mostly based on passion, emotion, and sex. We could go for hours, fight, have intercourse, embrace, and fight again. I seemed to pick women who could both fight and love. I was beginning to come alive, and was experiencing that rebirth in my sexual relationships and anger. I never considered myself a stud or woman's man. I was also serious minded, but short on commitment. She was artistic and had a matching, volatile disposition. Sexual sensations were also most likely substituting for drug effects for me. We could have sexual encounters that would last hours, interchanged with fury. A nice mix at the time. Other budding addictions to contend with, sex and anger.

Then, I made a fatal decision to play racquetball with

another woman. I can't say it was an innocent, platonic meeting. On the other hand, I didn't do anything that was sexual in nature. Anyway, my girlfriend went ballistic, threw me out of the house, said we were done. She went back to the relationship she had going on when I had originally met her. I was stunned; it happened so fast, no discussion, no second chances or reconsideration. Up to that point, our relationship had been rocky, and I didn't see it going anywhere long term, so I unconsciously severed my ties by meeting with the other woman.

Yet, I had a hard time letting go of that relationship, and had melancholy and longing for her long after she left me. She ignored my attempts to reconcile, and wanted nothing to do with someone she could not trust, according to her. My relationship with her ended for good. Lights out and plug pulled. Done and gone. Door cemented shut. I still think about her. I loved her passion. I still think about her.

Back to my residency, I never knew exactly what my Neurology Department thought of me but I didn't receive much negative feedback. We had some good residents so it wasn't like I didn't belong. Neurologists don't have particularly suave personalities, so maybe I just fit in at the time. I recall meeting with my Chair to discuss my interests in an academic position. He said I needed to develop a "stick" or specialty. I didn't know what that would be at that time, but I continued my fascination with drugs and entered a fellowship in Clinical Pharmacology. Pharmacology is the study of drugs and medications, particularly in humans. I met a very congenial mentor who set me up in the Fellowship in Clinical Pharmacology. I was still pretty self-directed, and pursued my own course in pharmacology. I spent two years learning about medications and other drugs.

At the same time, I moonlighted and worked as a

Neurologist for a large Neurology practice in Minneapolis. I worked on weekends and vacations providing consultations in Neurology. I was actually pretty good at it. Clinical Neurology was pretty logical and intuitive for me to understand. Eventuall I was offered a permanent job in the Neurology practice. But I was beginning to realize I was on a mission to work in addictions, and wanted to become a writer. I wanted to tell people about my experiences with alcohol and drugs, and to teach physicians.

I managed to complete my residency in Neurology from start to finish without an interruption, a first for me since high school. I had dropped out of college and medical school, internship, and residencies during my addiction days. Now I had found a way to abstain and stay sober in AA. I attributed most of it to not drinking and seeking guidance over and above me. Though I did have one incident that I thought might get me bounced where I angrily told an entitled resident to get "fucked," that was overheard by the chairman of her department. Just a chance passing in the hallway, unbelievably unlikely, but happened anyway. Nothing came of it and actually my Chair at the time told him my language was none of their business. Apparently, I was otherwise holding my own as a resident in the Department.

My life in AA was expanding and deepening. I was involved in "step work" increasingly. I now had reached the 4th and 5th Steps. Step 4: "Made a searching and fearless moral inventory of ourselves." Step 5: "Admit to God, to ourselves and to another human being the exact nature of our wrongs." The principles behind them are *Honesty, Self-Inventory, and Truth*—a confession of wrongs. Now I ask you, what does a moral inventory have to do with a disease, especially after I spent so much explanation. The short answer is I don't know, except addictive disease creates many moral issues that complicate our psyche and relationships. These moral issues are an expression of the addictive disease, and must be dealt with to recover and abstain, paradoxically.

A good rule of thumb for the inventory and confessions in Steps 4 and 5, are the seven cardinal sins for the basis of an inventory. Step 4: "Made a searching and fearless moral inventory of ourselves." Step 5: "Admitted to God, to ourselves, and to another human being the exact nature of our wrongs."

Step 4 is an inventory of how my instincts exceeded their proper function, and an effort to discover my liabilities. I had a disease of extremes in instinctive drives. A misguided, judgmental moral inventory can result in guilt, grandiosity, or blaming others. I also listed my assets with my noted, painful liabilities. I had buried my past wrongs in self-justification, a dangerous state. To start and complete my inventory, I had to have willingness and confidence to explore my past, and all its failings, as thoroughly as possible. Step 4 was the beginning of a lifetime, me practicing self-inventory. My common symptoms of emotional insecurity are fear, worry, anger, resentment, self-pity, and depression. My inventory reviews were based on relationships, and how my warped, emotional state and actions affected them. I had to be searching and fearless.

What confuses me to this day is that I believe alcoholism and drug addictions are physical, mental, and spiritual diseases. To me, addiction is a brain disease that leads to mental and spiritual consequences. There is ample science in animal and human studies to support addiction centers in the brain where compulsive drug and alcohol use originates and is sustained. I can also see, and science supports, where toxic effects of alcohol and drug use create and induce mental problems, such as depression, anxiety, and psychosis. And because alcohol and drug use forces one to behave and act in ways contrary to their moral or ethical codes, spiritual problems result, e.g. pride, sex, legal, interpersonal relationships.

However, just how does cleaning house and living in a way true to myself promote abstinence and recovery from drug addiction? We are admonished to be, "True to thyself," and not according to a religious or philosophical doctrine. It is the God of my understanding, an inventory by me, about me, and according to me, and not some other moral codes. However, general spiritual principles common to most, if not all recognized religions can be used as guides for fundamental human traits and characteristics.

Unfortunately, modern psychological and psychiatry deal more with the consequences than the origin of psychic disturbances. Medications and therapies cover up antecedent causes, and may even perpetuate psychic causes bv avoiding resolution. For instance, someone is anxious and depressed from feeling guilty about cheating on their spouse, and receives antidepressant medications without resolving the underlying causes. Avoiding the ethical dilemmas with medications will only prolong both the unacceptable behaviors and psychic disturbances. Finding balance with our conscience (a forgotten word), inner balance or karma, is the aim in Steps 4 and 5 to, strange as it may sound, avoid the first drink or drug. For us, to drink or drug is to suffer and perhaps die.

Thus, there are many conditions in ordinary life that lead to disturbances in mood, inner dissatisfaction, anger and resentments, not to mention a self-centered life. While I am not a proponent of sin, I do believe suggestions of sin do form a basis for a spiritual life. A list of seven sins that Christian God hates is found in 6:16-19 of the Bible: There are six things the Lord hates, seven that are detestable to him: "Haughty eyes, a lying tongue, hands that shed innocent blood, a heart that devises wicked schemes, feet that are quick to rush into evil, a false witness who pours out lies, and a man who stirs up dissension among brothers." While these character defects and shortcomings are religious in nature, they are also spiritual in practice. Acknowledgement and correction can make a big difference in continued abstinence from alcohol and drugs, and peace of mind and contentment.

The opposite for the 7 deadly sins are:

- *Chastity (purity) for Lust (undesired love)*
- *Moderation (self-restraint) for Gluttony (overindulgence)*
- *Generosity (vigilance) for Greed (avarice)*
- *Zeal (integrity) for Sloth (laziness)*
- *Meekness (composure) for Wrath (anger)*
- *Charity (giving) for Envy (jealousy)*
- *Humility (humbleness) for Pride (vanity)*

These opposites look like good orderly directions or general suggestions for spiritual development. In general, the more spiritually fit I become, the more likely I will refrain from relapse, and be helpful to others. A goal of spiritual development in AA according to the 12 Steps, is to carry the message to other alcoholics and drug addicts, and to be useful to others, not just addicts. A spiritual approach is a pragmatic approach, and most of us learn over time how to live a spiritual life. In *The Big Book of Alcoholics Anonymous'* chapter called "Spiritual Experience," it says,

William James called most of our experiences of the "educational variety," because they develop slowly over a period of time. Quite often friends of the newcomer are aware of the difference long before he is himself. He finally realizes that he has undergone a profound alteration in his reaction to life; that such a change could hardly have been brought about by himself alone. What often takes place in a few months could seldom have been accomplished by years of self-discipline. With few exceptions our members find that they have tapped an unsuspected inner resource, which they presently identify with their own conception of a Power greater than themselves...

We find that no one need have difficulty with the spirituality of the program. Willingness, honesty and open mindedness are the essentials of recovery. These are indispensable. "There is a principle which is a bar against all information, which is proof against all arguments and which cannot fail to keep a man in everlasting ignorance-that principle is contempt prior to investigation." —Herbert Spencer

In my 4th Step inventory, and that of others, certain character defects cannot be avoided if sobriety is to be expected. Trying to skip over them is fraught with danger and defeat in efforts to not drink, drug and to establish a commitment to recovery. *The Big Book of Alcoholics Anonymous* elaborates,

Resentment is the "number one" offender. It destroys more alcoholics than anything else. From it stems all forms of spiritual disease, for we have been not only mentally and physically ill, we have been spiritually sick. When the spiritual malady is overcome, we straighten out mentally and physically. In dealing with resentments, we set them on paper. We listed people, institutions or principles with whom we were angry. We asked ourselves why we were angry. In most cases it was out pocketbooks, our ambitions, our personal relationships (including sex) were hurt or threatened. So we were sore. We were "burned up." We went back through our lives. Nothing counted but thoroughness and honesty. When we were finished we considered it carefully. The first thing apparent was that this world and its people were often quite wrong. To conclude that others were wrong was as far as most of us ever got. The usual outcome was that people continued to wrong us and we stayed sore at ourselves. But the more we fought and tried to have it our own way, the worse matters got. As in war, the victor only seemed to win. Our moments of triumph were short-lived. It is plain that a life which includes deep resentment leads only to futility and unhappiness. To the precise extent that we permit these, do we squander the hours that might have been worthwhile. But with the alcoholic, whose hope is the maintenance and growth of a spiritual experience, this business of resentment is infinitely grave. We found that it is fatal. For when harboring such feelings we shut ourselves off the sunlight of the Spirit. The insanity of alcohol returns and we drink again. And with us, to drink is to die. If we were to live, we had to be free of anger. The grouch and the brainstorm were not for us. They may be the dubious luxury of normal men, but for the alcoholics these things are poison.

This short word (fear) somehow touches about every aspect of our lives. It was an evil and corroding thread: the fabric of our existence was shot through with it. It set in motion trains of circumstances which brought us misfortune we felt we didn't deserve. But did not we, ourselves, set the ball rolling? Sometimes we think fear ought to be classed with stealing. It seems to cause more trouble. We reviewed our fears thoroughly. We put them on paper, even though we had no resentment in connection with them. Wasn't it because self-reliance failed us? Self-reliance was good as far as it went, but it didn't go far enough. Some of us once had great self-confidence, but it didn't fully solve the fear problem, or any other. When it made us cocky, it was worse. Perhaps there is a better way- we think so. For we are now on a different basis: the basis of trusting and our finite selves. We are in the world to play the role He assigns. Just to the extent that we do as we think He would have us, and humbly rely on Him, does He enable us to match calamity with serenity.

We never apologize to anyone for depending upon our Creator. We can laugh at those who think spirituality the way of weakness. Paradoxically, it the way of strength. The verdict of the ages is that faith means courage. All men of faith have courage. They trust their God. We never apologize for God. Instead we let Him demonstrate, through us, what He can do. We ask Him to remove our fear and direct our attention to what He would have us be. At once we commence to outgrow fear.

I have taken several 4th and 5th Steps over the years. However, the first time I wanted an answer whether to leave Washington D.C. to move to Minnesota, my sponsor suggested I take a 4th Step. Not entirely sure why, I chose a fellow AA member in one of my groups for these steps. He seemed to have some sobriety, and a peacefulness about him. I made a list of how irresponsible I had become in my addictions, how many times I failed to meet expectations, and cited my dishonesty to others. I wasn't really aware of my fears and anger yet. I was pretty simple in this first fourth step. I don't know about you, but I am not particularly adept at seeing and identifying my emotions and understanding the exact nature of my wrongs. It wasn't until I had been sober awhile before I began to become aware of my feelings of anger. I had suppressed it for years. The new anger I felt was positive, the kind that supports survival and change. Anger as an instinct, which I used positively.

The 12 Steps deflated my bloated ego. Step 5 was particularly difficult but necessary to sobriety and peace of mind. Confession is an ancient discipline. Without fearless admission of defects, I could not stay sober. What did I receive from Step 5? I began a true kinship with man and God. I lost my sense of isolation, received forgiveness, and gave it. I learned humility, gained honesty and realism. I had to be completely truthful and sincere. And I had to avoid rationalization and choose a person in whom to confide. My results were a measure of tranquility and consciousness of God or a power greater than myself. Step 5: "Admit to God, to ourselves, and to another human being the exact nature of our wrong."

Fear is a natural reaction to confession. Although I may want recovery desperately, the thought of revealing my innermost, personal self to another human being may be terrifying. If I allowed these feelings to stop my progress at step five, I would stop moving forward in my recovery and the disease of alcohol addiction will take over once more. Alcoholics Anonymous Step 4 prepared me for Step 5, and by finding the courage to overcome that fear of rejection or the shame of my confession, I experienced honesty on a deeper level than my first step of admission.

I broke the pattern of denial that often plagues those suffering with addictions. Step 5 strengthened this foundation and reaffirmed my commitment to recovery. In Alcoholic's Anonymous' book *Twelve Steps and Twelve Traditions* it states:

If we skip this vital step, we may not overcome drinking. Time after time newcomers have tried to keep to themselves certain facts about their lives. Trying to avoid this humbling experience, they have turned to easier methods. Almost invariably they got drunk. Having persevered with the rest of the program, they wondered why they fell. We think the reason is that they never completed their housecleaning. They took inventory all right, but hung on to some of the worst items in stock. They only thought they had lost their egoism and fear; they only thought they had humbled themselves. But they had not learned enough of humility, fearlessness and honesty, in the sense we find it necessary, until they told someone else their life story.

I took several 5th Steps over the years with AA sponsors and Clergy. Each time I had the satisfaction of completion but not miraculous relief. I gained confidence in my ability to remain sober each time. Taking action is the heart and soul of my spiritual discovery and recovery from addictions. I learned over time about my resentments or fears or wrongs or guilt that fueled my drinking. And that I could do something about my sorry mental and emotional states. I could reduce my judgmental attitude, and could separate myself from my guilt and shame.

Guilt is responsibility for doing something bad or wrong. A bad feeling caused by knowing or thinking against my conscience. Shame is feeling guilt, regret, or sadness that I am bad, not just knowing I have done something wrong. Shame is a dangerously painful emotion caused by consciousness of guilt, shortcoming, or impropriety. A condition of humiliating disgrace or dispute, something that brings censure or reproach, something to be regretted. Shame is not conducive to recovery, rather more likely to promote relapse and self-destruction.

The shame condemned me, and drove me to suicide, defeat, personal bankruptcy in drinking, and would do the same in abstinence. I lived in a black cloud, threatening to eliminate me unless I continued to take actions in the steps. Each 5th step lessened my shame, but not all at once by just talking to someone and God. I recall confession with a Catholic Priest who wanted to know all about my masturbations, when, how many times. But confession did not end my masturbation, and confession just increased my guild and shame, not reduced it.

However, my wrongs admitted in the Step 5 were lessened because I shared with another person who understood me and my purpose, and a God who potentially forgave me and more importantly helped me to forgive myself. Shame was my biggest challenge, an overwhelming negative judgment of myself, by myself and for myself. Revealing my sources of shame helped me to redeem myself, value myself and end my self-destructive acts. But work remained.

Even though I was making progress in getting my emotions under control, I was still attracted to volcanoes. I met another woman, again attractive and passionate, but not realistic for me from the start. She had 3 children, worked as nurse, and was recently divorced. She was definitely charming and vivacious. We made love on our first date as she captured me in the kitchen. Our mutual personal and sexual passions kept us together for a while until my future changed. She had a history of drama like my other passionate relationships. I got caught up in that, and God did I crave it. These sexual encounters with passionate and beautiful women definitely helped me come alive, experience pleasure I had not experienced, perhaps ever, and supplied energy to move forward in my spiritual awakening.

As I told you, I never believed that I had a relationship with God where he, she, or it would intervene in my life. I always was good at asking God for things, but was never convinced He could, or would do anything. But after I did Step 3, a power greater than myself was working in my life and I *was* staying sober. After I worked Steps 4 and 5, I was realizing I was consulting God regularly on my mission. The Blues Brothers and the Band. Jake and Elwood had every good intention of paying the back taxes for the orphanage. Elwood said they were on a mission from God, as I was, and still am today. I had seen the light, I was in the band, and I had begun my mission from God.

"Yes, yes! Jesus H. goddamned bastard Christ,
I have seen the light!"

—The Blues Brothers (1980), Director John Landis

10

MY MISSION FROM GOD

*"Even if you're on the right track, you'll get
run over if you just sit there."* —Will Rogers

I experienced the strangest sensations while in Minnesota.
I found I could not look people in the eye. People I didn't
know, had never met and had no prior dealings with. I
was very uncomfortable in a place where I had never lived
nor done damage, or had personal experiences. I was overwhelmed with shame and guilt. I am uncertain why it took
so long for my past to erupt and intrude on my present. I
had been sober for several months. I must say, leaving a
residency abruptly didn't help my state of mind, but the
agony extended beyond.

I knew I had a remorseful past, but did not know how
much it affected me. After about a year of carrying around
the albatross of my transgressions, having taken the 4th and
5th Steps, I faced the daunting task of becoming ready to be
relieved of my shame and guilt. First, I had to become willing to be relieved of the self-centeredness, anger, resentments, guilt, shame, intolerance, and impatience, which
plagued me. Step 6 provided a mechanism for God, or my
Higher Power, to remove these emotional time bombs and
painful memories from my consciousness, and particularly,
unconsciousness. If I cannot face strangers because of my
past, I have a poor prognosis for living in the present and

future, and ultimately staying sober.

As surmountable obstacles, I learned through AA I possessed character defects that were causing me suffering and shortcomings that were interfering with my attitudes and relationships. Steps 6 and 7 provided a way to find more self-acceptance and dedication to a reliance on spiritual power. I started to learn how to help others, becoming a priority in my career and life. I learned over time that I could stay sober and change by helping others with drug and alcohol problems, through my work. I became willing to change and asked God for help no matter how little humility I may have had at the time. I did not understand fully what character defects and shortcomings had to do with becoming a better doctor or friend. I certainly still blamed others for my feelings and actions, and wanted to change them rather than change me.

Alcoholics Anonymous Step 6 says, "We're entirely ready to have God remove all these defects of character," and that, "We became willing to ask God to help us remove our defects of character." To understand exactly how this step works and what you need to do to take it, you may need to think about the steps that came before it. I started by admitting I was powerless over alcohol and that my life had become unmanageable; I could not control my drinking, came to believe that a power greater than myself could, made a decision to use that power, and looked and admitted to myself, someone else, and God especially, the wreckage of my past.

I certainly had to be entirely ready to have God remove all my defects of character in Step 6, Although I grew up in an angry and resentful environment, I was not accustomed to or attracted to anger ordinarily. However, I had acquired a great amount of anger in my addiction days, and emerged with fury. I like to explain it like inflammation, red, tender, hot, and sensitive, an exposed feeling. In my early recovery I had very few normal feelings other than pain and suffering, as I withdrew from the drugs, Valium and Darvon. Vice like headaches, gripping sensations, intolerable tension, dark days, unable to visualize my thoughts, or identify any particular emotions, feeling flooded and numb. I had a sign in my room, "This too shall pass," that I looked at every day because I felt so miserable my first two years of sobriety. I literally could only barely make it one day at a time.

Here I was, also a resident working 90-100 hours a week, adding to my misery, living on fatigue and sometimes little sleep. My first emotion I could identify was anger, anger that persists to this day. Maybe some of that is characterological from my parents who reacted to life with anger at times. After all, my father was a fighter, not a lover. My mother was both.

Now what in God's name do I do with the admitted shame, guilt, and resentments? Remained condemned to life with, "No Exit," as Sartre suggested? Live in the Inferno as Dante proclaimed? Or just suffer as the existentialist Camus tells us? Just disclosing them to myself and others is not enough. I had to find a way to dump them, and get rid of them. Somehow, I had to become entirely ready to it. How in the hell could I become entirely ready? I can't remember any time in my life where I was entirely ready to do anything! Honesty, openness, willingness are the keys. Just the opposite of what I had done up to this point. I had lied to myself, others and tried to completely forget about God.

Before getting to this point, I first had to admit that I had an alcohol and drug problem, explore the concept of higher power, and begin developing a relationship with that higher power. I also had to look honestly at my shortcomings and myself so that I could get ready to ask God to remove them. So, this challenging step, which is the culmination of all the work I had done beforehand, asks the alcoholic and drug addict to admit that he is powerless over all of his negative behavior, not just his drinking, and consider turning these behaviors over to his higher power. This can be scary or embarrassing just like when the alcoholic admitted he was powerless over alcohol. However, the step didn't ask to turn over your defects yet—it just asks you to become *willing* to do so.

After I had more or less successfully completed the first six steps of the 12 Steps of Alcoholics Anonymous, I was ready to move on to AA Step 7. In Steps 3 through 6, I had made the decision to turn my will and my life over to "God as I had understood Him," tackled the task of making a "searching and fearless moral inventory" of myself, admitted my wrongs, and was "entirely ready" to let God remove my defects. In the 7th Step of Alcoholics Anonymous, I humbly asked "Him to remove my shortcomings." In order to compete this task successfully, I needed to understand what it meant to be truly humble.

Understanding and learning humility is not an easy or natural task for me. My addictions and even my personality were grandiose and self-righteous. Drunk or sober, I gravitated towards self-justification and rationalization. To get a good grasp on the concept of humility, try picturing circumstances in your life (real or imagined), where humility comes into play and determine how being humble can influence your interaction with God as you understand Him while working through AA Step 7.

One definition of humility is to be "not proud or arrogant; modest." This example of humility is a lesson learned early in life. Imagine yourself as a kindergartner who just created the most beautiful picture of a bunny any kindergartner had ever seen. At least that's how you felt when your teacher complimented your drawing and held it up in front of the class. Immediately, you were filled with the natural response of pride.

At that point, you would have transitioned from natural pride to either modest pride or arrogant pride. The choice was yours whether you were conscious of it or not. Modest pride would have filled you with the good feeling of accomplishing something special; arrogant pride would have filled you with that same feeling with the added sense of *feeling superior* to your kindergarten peers. So, to be truly humble, you would have stopped at the natural pride before allowing it to make you feel superior. Therein lies the difference between arrogance and humility: proportionate pride vs. disproportionate pride, collegiality vs. superiority, realistic vs. distorted reality, open vs. closed to facts.

Step 7: "Humbly asked Him to remove our shortcomings," meant I had to ask God or my Higher Power to remove my resentments, shame, guilt, and pride. I can't really explain just how to do that to you. You see this is one of the steps where I "act as if" and see what happens. The key is that I give up trying to remove my shortcomings on my own, that I seek a greater power, seek a spiritual solution to my personality problems, and most importantly I humbled myself enough to ask for help. Not a natural or easy step for me. Not a joy ride, but the results are stupendous and life saving. Out of a self-imposed prison of shame and guilt, darkness, futility, and into freedom, light, and hope. Yet, I still could not look people in the eye. I still was filled with shame and guilt. I still had more work to do. Time to get off my knees and pick up the hoe and start to take actions. I had to do something.

My father started it off. He called me after a year of not drinking and drugging. He wanted to know how I was doing. He had heard I was not drinking. I confirmed I was now in a residency for Neurology at the University of Minnesota. I had not called him during that year. He opened up a world of possibilities. I instinctively knew if I was going to stay alive, I had to complete Steps 8 and 9, and make amends to the world I had trashed and left behind. I had to face the path of destruction that had tried to kill me, and still had the capability to do so. I intuitively realized I must become willing to make amends and actually make amends to those I had harmed due to my drinking and drug addictions. Starting with myself.

I began to make amends at places where I had done damage in my career. I had established quite a path of destruction, lost relationships, missed opportunities, humiliation, and embarrassment. I learned that I was making amends to myself while I was making amends to others. I was number one on any list of atonements. You have to understand, what I did to myself, the shame I carried around like a heavy noose, caused me to avoid contact with people. Shame was to me, condemnation and judgments of myself, by myself, for myself.

I had become alienated from society, family, friends, colleagues, just about everyone. I saw myself as superior to all other people and so could not relate to anyone. I saw other people as tools and used them for my own ends. As my addiction worsened over time, my isolation grew because of my intense guilt and the delirium from my regular use of intoxicating drugs and alcohol, with its consequent guilt. Over and over again, I pushed away the people trying to help me, and suffered the consequences from further alienation. In the end, I found the total isolation that I brought upon myself intolerable. When I finally started to list those I had harmed in Step 8, and began to actually make amends in Step 9, I broke through the wall of pride and self-centeredness that had separated me from society.

My inner world with all of its doubts, deliria, second-guessing, fear, and despair, is the heart of my story of addiction. My recovery through the steps forced me to deal with tormenting guilt. Any actual punishment I received as a result of my addiction was much less terrible than the stress and anxiety of trying to avoid punishment. Because I necessarily experienced great mental torture, I understood as a guilt-ridden alcoholic and addict, I must eventually confess to others the exact nature of my wrongs and make amends. Otherwise, go mad or relapse to alcohol and drugs. I could not escape the natural outcomes of my addictions.

I became grandiose, paradoxically in my increasing self-depreciation from my ever-worsening addictions. I considered myself at times as a "superman," a person who is extraordinary and thus above the moral rules that govern the rest of humanity. My vaunted estimation of myself compelled me to separate myself from society. My inability to quell my subsequent feelings of guilt, however, proved to me that I was not a "superman."

Although I realized my failure to live up to what I had envisioned for myself, I was nevertheless unwilling to accept the total deconstruction of my addictive identity. I continued to resist the idea that I was as mediocre as the rest of humanity by maintaining that my addictive use of drugs and alcohol were justified. It is only in my surrender of my ego and pride in the steps, that I realized the release of guilt and the joys in such surrender, that I finally escaped my conception of myself as a superman and the terrible isolation such a belief brought upon me.

My redemption which began in Steps 4 and 5 by identifying the sources of my mental anguish, and continued in Steps 6 and 7 to become willing and humble to have my mental anguish removed, was now on the brink of release; the beginning of the end and a return to society. Up to then I had denied any conscious feeling of sin or devoutness even after I had admitted my wrongs, and not yet achieved redemption or even understood what amends could offer me. But I had begun on the path toward recognition of the wrongs I had committed and sources of my guilt and shame. I now look forward to the journey to beginning of the end and to humanity. And like that of Jesus, according to Christianity, I will ultimately be saved and renewed.

Faced with the humiliation of defeat and the suffering, I began to examine many of his questions about existence with respect to my life of addiction. I was living in hell occupied by myself (who I could not stand), as divided into three people in my id, superego, and ego. The id drove my addictive use of alcohol drugs, the superego condemned its use, and ego kept failing to find a way to control the chaos and confusion. I examined such issues as freedom, self-deception, and the nature of time in my pursuit of listing and making amends.

Throughout my whole story and recovery, I looked back to the past and to the present, trying to make peace with myself about the evil things I had done to loved ones and not so loved ones. Guilt and shame ruled my life for many years during my addiction, now I painstaking faced my anguish head on. I had made a decision to live, and had to find a way out of my living hell or die. I had to learn to live in the here and now. I had to forgive the past, and face the future, the two most dangerous places for me. I had to accept the present without fear and trembling or drink or drug, which for me was to die. Living in the present was my exit from my hell.

As I was making amends, I realized I was carrying the message for recovery in AA as explained by my purpose and recovery. As I returned from making amends, I was able to face people more directly without shame in Minnesota. I started to feel God was doing for me what I could not do for myself, and I felt a great uplift and euphoria. I had my spiritual experience and communion with a force greater than myself.

Steps 8 and 9 are concerned with personal relations. Learning to live with others was a daunting adventure for me. Up to that point, the obstacles were reluctance to forgive, not admitting my wrongs to other, purposeful and drug induced forgetting. From my exhaustive survey of past, and deepening insight results from my thorough inventory of the kinds of harm done to others. While avoiding extreme judgment, I had taken an objective view through Step 8 which was the beginning of the end of isolation.

Step 8: "Made a list of all persons we had harmed, and became willing to make amends to them all." So, I looked over my personal inventory in Steps 4, 5, 6, 7 and possibly reflected on my life again. I made a list of the people that I had harmed. My test was if I thought or felt I had harmed them and to discuss with my sponsors. I wrote down thoughts beside each name about what the appropriate amends might be. I then went through the list and made sure I was entirely willing in my heart to make the amends.

My family came first, prior relationships, and my medical education and training were listed, where I had spent so much of my life. I had little trouble listing them, and found as I made amends, I generated a longer list, and enthusiasm to make more amends. I loved the freedom from my mental anguish; it was an adventure to depart from my hell. The guiding principal of this step is to make full amends at the earliest opportunity, as long as such action is feasible, proper, and will not cause additional harm. *Twelve Steps and Twelve Traditions* tells us,

Learning how to live in the greatest peace, partnership and brotherhood with all men and women, of whatever description, is a moving and fascinating adventure. Every AA has found that he can make little headway in this new adventure of living until he first backtracks and really makes an accurate and unsparing survey of the human wreckage he has left in his wake. To a degree, he has already done this when taking moral inventory, but now the time has come when he ought to redouble his efforts to see how many people he has hurt, and in what ways. This reopening of emotional wounds, some old, some perhaps forgotten, and some still painfully festering, will at first look like a purposeless and pointless piece of surgery. But if a willing start is made, then the great advantages of doing this will so quickly reveal themselves that the pain will be lessened as one obstacle after another melts away.

In Step 9 I had to be willing to go to any lengths to make amends. "Made direct amends to such people wherever possible, except when to do so would injure them or others." I must be willing to take this step no matter how severe the personal consequences. If making amends required me to report a past crime, I must be willing to go to jail to complete this step on the road to recovery. The spiritual aspect of the mandates encouraged me in recovery to seek strength and guidance to do the right thing from a higher power and from the others engaged in the AA program.

I began with Johns Hopkins Department of Psychiatry where I had overdosed on drugs, and had my life saved. I met with the Chair of the Department who accepted me warmly, though he understood little about alcoholism. Also, I met with my past Residency Director, who agreed to have me return to finish my residency. I met with one faculty member who said he did not want to be part of my recovery program, though he didn't explain why. Some staff members hugged me and said they knew about my problem. Overall, I was well-received and shown love and respect. I left with euphoria and elevated spirits, as if I had been on a mission from God, which to me, I had.

My message had been short and simple. I confessed I was an alcoholic and drug addict, and claimed responsibility for my past drunken and drugged behaviors, and informed them I had established recovery in Alcoholics Anonymous. While my explanation had been accepted, I was not questioned. The Department and Johns Hopkins offered me readmission to complete my residency but I declined because I had established a life in Minnesota, so I thought.

After my father had called me to ask how I was doing, I made a visit to him in Florida. During our visit, he stunned me by saying I should continue to go to AA. He was happy that I had found a way to abstain from alcohol and drugs. In my life, I felt he had been a very judgmental person, who had said I lacked push, shove, and drive. After I admitted I was an alcoholic, he was not judgmental and did not think joining AA was a sign of weakness. It also was one of the few actions I took that he supported in my lifetime, and was life-saving.

Curiously, I met with my mother who had seen me on a ventilator in the intensive care unit at Johns Hopkins.

Surprisingly, she asked if I wanted a drink, I had to refuse of course. Alcohol was cunning, baffling, and powerful, and I had to be ever vigilant if a mother who loved me, offered me the very poison that almost killed me. After making amends, I began to experience the AA's 12 promises from *The Big Book of Alcoholics Anonymous*:

1. *We are going to know a new freedom and a new happiness.*
2. *We will not regret the past nor wish to shut the door on it.*
3. *We will comprehend the word serenity.*
4. *We will know peace.*
5. *No matter how far down the scale we have gone, we will see how our experience can benefit others.*
6. *The feelings of uselessness and self-pity will disappear.*
7. *We will lose interest in selfish things and gain interest in our fellows.*
8. *Self-seeking will slip away.*
9. *Our whole attitude and outlook on life will change.*
10. *Fear of people and economic insecurity will leave us.*
11. *We will intuitively know how to handle situations which used to baffle us*
12. *We will suddenly realize that God is doing for us what we could not do for ourselves.*

"Are these extravagant promises? We think not. They are being fulfilled among us—sometimes quickly, sometimes slowly. They will always materialize if we work for them."

I now had reestablished connections to my past and began to build my personal and professional future. I knew a new freedom. I was now creating foundations of recovery to chart a course to help myself by helping others. I now had to learn how to support my mission and be a mercenary. I had to get a job.

I was about eight years into my recovery and was now ready to carry the message even further. I had completed residencies in Neurology and Psychiatry, and passed board certification in Neurology and board certification in Electroencephalography (monitoring electrical activity of the brain). The next step was to launch an academic career. I asked myself with whom would I want to establish my academic career? While contemplating in my small cubicle office in Clinical Pharmacology, I asked what it was I wanted to do in my career and life? The answer was, "To learn how to write and write, write, write." Next inspiration was how, whom, when.

Not long after, I thought of Ronald Blake MD, a world famous academic writer in alcoholism. He wrote many books and journal articles. He had done valuable research in genetics of alcoholism. His adoption studies at the University of Copenhagen in Denmark showed alcoholism in biological parents of adoptees, and non-adoptees raised in an alcoholic environment, which ultimately predicted alcoholism in male adoptees. In other words, genetic background, and not environment, was responsible for development of alcoholism.

Dr. Blake was himself a notorious alcoholic, but was still admired and valued for his research and writings. I knew about his alcoholism before I interviewed. I dropped by his office to ask for a job, and he said yes. I was on a mission, and I wanted to save him along the way. Up to this point in my life, I had never shown an interest in writing, avoiding it like the plague.

The next thing I knew I was in my car driving to Kansas City, leaving my girlfriend behind again. I had purchased a BMW 320i. I continuously played albums by Phil Collins and Genesis, who had become my heartbeat, listening to them in the car, or while running and jogging everywhere. Leaving Minnesota was a terribly hard decision, as I had established a solid recovery in the Mecca of AA in Minnesota, bought a home, and was in a romantic and sexual relationship with a nurse I had met in one of the hospitals in Minnesota.

After I arrived in Kansas City, I noted Dr. Blake's active alcoholism while working in his Department of Psychiatry. I used his mentorship to start to write, but I never caught on the research in a big way. The purpose of research in Medical Schools then and still now, is to get big government grants. Research itself and results were not as important or valued. The goal of research is to create questions to apply for more money to support jobs, and universities. I was interested in knowledge and showing what worked and finding conclusions. I wanted to tell the world about alcoholism, and later drug addiction to help others. I had found solutions and ways to abstain from alcoholism, and wanted to share them. I learned the best way to stay sober and develop spiritually was to "carry the message" to those still suffering from addictions.

While in Kansas City, I had met yet another woman,

quite a bit younger than I. She had an irresistible look in her eyes about her. We started dating, and began having passionate sexual marathons. She was pretty exciting. She had a boyfriend back home in Minnesota as I had a girl-friend there too. She was pretty advanced and thought I was pretty "good" in arousing her sexual responses. She initially recommended me to someone else, but I declined, as I liked her.

I started to work for the Kansas State Medical Board. I spent a day intervening and confronting doctors who had alcohol and drug problems that had come to the attention of the medical board. I approached them with my rigorous mission to push them into treatment and recovery with the hammering power of the medical board. Also, with other doctors, I had founded the organization, *Physician Serving Physicians*, which worked with doctors referred by the Minnesota Medical Society to assist them in entering treatment and recovery. My mission to save the world was gaining steam and momentum.

I found however, that carrying the message would become a rocky path filled with pitfalls, obstacles, joy, success, sadness, and defeat. In my sincere effort to intervene, I approached the Dean of Kansas Medical School about Dr. Blake's alcoholism, in an effort to help save the life of a valuable academician. The Dean was not impressed by my efforts and must have told him about it. The next thing I knew I was the target of an inquisition.

I was performing electro-convulsive therapy (ECT) on a patient, when two faculty members alleged my technique lacking because I did not use electroencephalogram (EEG) recordings properly during ECT. Mind you, I was board certified in EEG and Neurology at the time. However, I was reported to the credentialing committee. I had no due process. The inquisition was meant to cover up and chill my efforts with Dr. Blake's alcoholism. I later found out that they were protecting more than that however, as he was removed from his position in the medical school because he was found guilty of embezzlement. He later died of a "heart attack." Or maybe alcoholism. After all, it's not a cause of death that is often made public. I had not succeeded in my mission with him. But God had Dr. Blake bequeath his knowledge of writing to me before he died. He had terminated my position in the Department soon after I tried to intervene to save his life from his eventual death from alcoholism. On to my next mission, or so I thought.

Just before I left Kansas, I met Dr. Scott Kirby at a medical conference, and asked him for a job on the spot. He responded by offering me a position at Fair Oaks Hospital in Summit NJ. So I moved to Nyack, New York, just outside of New York City, to commute to Summit. At the time, Dr. Kirby was one of the most famous doctors in the world who was doing research and publishing on cocaine and other drug addictions. He was a magic potion and rocket booster for my writing career. I began doing some research in family history of drug addiction as a carryover from my work with Dr. Blake. But the thrust was to write, and as usual I did it addictively, with drive and compulsivity.

I joined The American Society of Addiction Medicine, and gave talks and conferences. The first published book I edited, a comprehensive handbook on drug and alcohol addiction, won an award from the American Writer's Association. It was a masterpiece, if I say so myself, and the first of its kind. The book came together very naturally for me. Up to this point, I had been mentored by two of the most famous authors and researchers in the addiction and psychiatry fields, and perhaps the world, Dr. Blake and Dr.

Kirby, and it showed in my productivity and work. My list of publications grew, grew, and grew.

However, my occupation outside of academia didn't last long. In an unusual move, I chose to leave the position, instead of being escorted out, and accept an academic position with The New York Hospital Cornell Medical Center, Westchester Division, where I became the Head of the Alcohol Treatment Unit. There I established credentials as an Ivy Leaguer. I didn't make a whole lot of money, but I did gain fame and credibility as I learned how to treat clinical addicts and alcoholics.

But once again I took a hard line position with the Chair of Psychiatry, that I did not want to turn the Alcohol and Drug Unit into a Dual Diagnosis Unit, or rather, treating psychiatric patients with alcohol and drug problem. I told him he could find someone else. I had wanted to leave to return to the Midwest anyway. He sent me packing by what was to become a familiar theme of nonrenewal of contract. I stood by my principles and lost ground again. I remained determined to treat addiction as a primary disease, and wanted to work in a more medical environment. It would not be the last time I would lose a battle over addictions in an academic setting.

Please give me one more night
'Cause I can't wait forever

—"One More Night" Phil Collins

11

FATE

"Do What Thy Manhood Bids Thee To Do."
—Sir Richard Burton

I didn't know it yet but I was about to meet a woman who would change my life forever, for better or worse. I had planned to make another trip to Europe in search of the future mother of my children, so I thought. I had mapped out the countries I would visit next for my excursion. On my first trip I recall, as I lifted off from the airport in France I saw on a map in the airline magazine, and decided I would return to Germany. I can't tell you how or why I chose Germany, it was as if a power inserted its will for me, and later instilled the power to carry it out.

Perhaps, my status as a second-generation immigrant called me to my strong connection to my heritage. I had grown up with people who spoke broken English, or little English at all. Both grandmothers had not fully mastered English after coming from the "old country."

No offense, but I really didn't feel comfortable with American women. They did not hold the mystery or the fury I was looking for. The Swiss psychiatrist Carl Jung had a theory of the Collective Unconscious whereby our behavior is influenced and directed by ancestral drives and experiences. My attraction to Europe, and the Old Country was an unconscious drive to reconnect with my past to continue it into the future.

Furthermore, only one side of my family was educated to the extent they had graduated from high school and college. I was the second of the immigrant migration to graduate from college and the first to graduate from professional or graduate school. I had prepared myself for this trip, and needed time to build a foundation in my career before I could take on the next chapter in my journey, in my mission from God.

After I was run out of Kansas City for my bold acts to "help others," I landed in a familiar historical place for me, New York. My father's side of the family had immigrated to New York, through Ellis Island. To this day I am uncertain if my surname had been given to them at birth or while passing through immigration to shorten their Romanian and Polish Jewish names. My surname is a Polish name so I could have a genuine ancestral label. They landed in the Bronx for some reason, and I recall visiting my Romanian Grandmother in her small apartment near the Grand Concourse. I also had relatives who lived on Long Island.

Ironically I had been afraid of the big city, and always had stayed clear of the Big Apple. But this time felt different, I was on a mission from God, and so my grandiosity took over. I wanted to become famous and spread the word as I knew it and was coming to know it. I wanted to qualify to the world that I had found the power I had so sorely lacked in my addictions. I wanted them to know and to share with them what I had discovered.

I found a place to live in Nyack, New York, a town on the Hudson River just 20-30 minutes north of New Jersey and the George Washington Bridge to Manhattan. When I lived there, it maintained its simple, rustic charm. Nyack was the home of the famous actress, Helen Hayes, whose majestic house was on the Hudson near town and hospital named after her. Another claim to fame was as the birthplace and site for Edward Hopper's art collection. I am a fan, and have had one of his pictures hung in my office for most of my career. The town itself had no chain stores, but instead had second hand shops, worn bars, and no hotels I can remember. It did have a hospital and college, and many trees that lined the streets.

Nyack reminded me of a chapter out of the past, nothing like the upscale, modern cities on the other side of the Hudson in Westchester County. I am not sure Nyack had a distinction or commerce beyond its shipbuilding days, and its sparse population and surroundings reflected chosen limited economic resources. I can't explain why the Rockland County side of the Hudson had not kept pace with the cosmopolitan New York area. And why a train had not been constructed to connect the Rockland side of the Hudson River. The lack of a train, and modern transportation beyond bus service and the Henry Hudson Parkway, explained why the area remained a thing of the past. The population had grown only to 500 since 1990 when I lived there, from 6,500 to 7,000 people. A virtual island 19 miles north of Manhattan on the West side of the Hudson.

I still had to commute via the New York State Thruway and New Jersey Turnpike to Summit, New Jersey, the home of the Fair Oaks Hospital and the famous Dr. Scott Kirby. I started working on an addiction/detoxification unit, learning firsthand how to detoxify patients from drugs and alcohol, and to behaviorally treat their addictive drive to use compulsively. I participated in groups, and had a stern taskmaster who oversaw care and led groups with an iron hand. He controlled not only the patients but also me. He noted immediately that I was different from other doctors because I had a certain humility about me. I revealed my anonymity as a recovering alcoholic and drug addict. But to him that did not constitute treatment, and continuously reigned me into my place in the treatment process. Eventually, I was able to lead my own group on the first step, about powerlessness and unmanageability over alcohol and drugs. He led the more sophisticated stuff about how to change and live without alcohol and drugs.

I started to write articles with Dr. Kirby. He was brilliant and simple. He distilled his ideas into a few sentences, and did not devote a lot of time and energy to analysis and explanation. I recall we discussed addiction, and I gave him my three prongs of addictive behaviors: preoccupation, compulsivity, and relapse. He blurted out, "You don't need more than preoccupation," with acquiring alcohol and drugs. I pondered and agreed that probably is all you need to identify addictive behavior, but think continued use in spite of adverse consequences as in compulsivity is what confirms addictive use. He gave me the observation that many cocaine addicts use alcohol, and the two reinforced the use of the other.

Explanations were, some cocaine addicts were alcoholics before trying cocaine, that alcohol enhanced the effects of cocaine and treated the jittery consequences of heavy use of stimulants; to come down from the sustained high from cocaine. I reviewed admissions from years past, and started keeping track of the known admissions for the concurrent use of cocaine and alcohol, and found a very high correlation. I found multiple drug addictions to be the rule rather than the exception. And I published these findings in medical journals. I can't say I won the Nobel Prize, but I began to make contributions to the field, and to the understanding drug addictions.

From my work with Dr. Ronald Blake, I applied my interest in family history and genetics to cocaine addiction. I did not have a grant or use fancy methods, but asked simple questions like, "Do you have family members," preferably, biologically related members, "with drug and alcohol addiction?" I found an astounding prevalence among related family members for drug and alcohol addiction in my cocaine patients, just as the family history studies for alcohol. More observations implied that drug and alcohol addictions had a genetic basis and did not originate out of character or misunderstandings and bad breaks. I published those findings as well in medical journals. I thought everyone was interested in these self-evident truths, no matter what.

The call of academia, my desire to teach, and to have a bully pulpit so to speak, was strong. The New York Hospital Cornell University Medical College, Westchester Division, advertised a position in the New York Times for a Unit Chief of an Alcohol and Drug Unit. I applied. I always wanted to be an Ivy Leaguer, so this was my chance.

The Westchester Division was in White Plains, New York, in Westchester County. I would commute from Nyack across the Tappen Zee Bridge on the New State Thruway. I did not get the position right away. The Chair of the Department of Psychiatry in the Cornell University Medical College did not approve my appointment, despite my obvious clinical qualifications. So I agreed to come on as a temporary appointment to take away their risks if I turned out to be dud.

After several months, and with the help of my staff, I convinced them to hire me into a permanent position as the Unit Chief. I had inherited a unit with a psychiatric focus, low admission rates, and without leadership. Within a year I had the unit running in full, training staff, and implementing treatment programs for addictions. A nurse stepped up and developed marvelous detoxification protocols for the patients, and provided great clinical leadership on the unit for the staff. We had a social worker who inspired us all with her expertise in families and addictions. I learned from her if an addict was balking in treatment it was because of a relationship that was pulling them out of treatment. Often the same relationship that supported and propelled their addictions.

You understand I had always wanted a family, so I then began my search for a wife in earnest. I had been in multiple, mostly short-term relationships, unable to commit myself to long-term bondage as I thought. I was also accustomed to taking the difficult road and doing things the hard way. So, I got on a plane to Germany. I landed in Frankfort, and attended an AA meeting that was conducted in German language exclusively. I remember seeing an AA Big Book written in German at the meeting. I don't remember if I shared verbally, but I could feel the spirit of the meeting and the tone of recovery.

I had a routine of running or jogging through cities in Europe and the U.S. on the streets and sidewalks. I enjoyed stopping at cafés for coffee, licorice, and chocolate. I ran in shorts and tank top, and visited museums, particularly, art museums in Munich, Venice, and Vienna. I could tour a city in hours as opposed to days, see the people on the street, and view the gardens. I could run with these interludes for the days and nights. I would feel the runner's glow and euphoria, relaxing me. I was able to save up my money from not using taxis. I had always dreamed of driving on the Autobahn, so I drove a BMW from Frankfort to Vienna, Austria, back to Munich.

Don't ask me how I had planned this trip because

I can't tell you. I just outlined countries I wanted to see. I knew nothing about Europe, and picked hotels out of the blue. I had some unwavering trust that European cities were safe, and I could travel without fear from city to city and country to country.

Vienna was spectacular. It had two distinct lives, the inner circle of the old neighborhoods from Pre World War II and the outer circle of newer neighborhoods from Post War. The inner circle was old and historic, and the outer was modern and without the same character. I could imagine the symphony concerts by the great composers and conductors such as Mozart. I drove back to Munich on the Autobahn, and remember cars whizzing by me at over 100 miles an hour. Munich was a truly post war city; quite modern, and not much in the way of history to see. A good deal of the city had been bombed during WWII, and replaced with contemporary architecture. It was pleasant but not overly cultural. My next destination was Zurich, Switzerland. Don't ask me why again. Destiny, I think.

As I boarded the train in the Munich train station for Zurich, I saw two open seats next to young women. I had a choice between a well-dressed attractive, American looking woman, and an equally dressed, attractive, but very European looking woman. I chose the latter instinctively, not knowing why again. She wore simple clothes, no makeup, and natural hair. As I started a conversation with her, I realized she spoke limited English. She understood me more than I understood her. Yet we talked most of the trip through the beautiful Swiss mountains, in my unfolding idyllic, romantic adventure. I barely could communicate with her but we pursued each other, nonetheless. The look is greater than the word, the dream is greater than the reality, and the desire is greater than the logic.

We started to talk about addiction after I told her what I did for a living. She told me about the food addiction she had been struggling with. She had other addictions as well. We talked continuously, though not fluently. She was 23 and I was 44 at the time. Her age seemed ideal to me for my purpose of having a family and my youthful emotions, given my addictions through my early adulthood. I had matched her emotional immaturity, and as I would later find out, rage as well.

We arranged to meet for dinner in Zurich, and she brought her brother, which was somewhat disappointing for me, as I had wanted a more romantic rendezvous, but encouraging nonetheless. She had told me about her father's explosive, angry, and destructive moods, but I didn't think for a moment she was talking about herself in a way too.

After spending only a few hours with her, I invited her to visit me in the U.S. in Nyack. She said she would get back with me later. Not doubting her, she called to say she accepted my invitation. Back then we had no working Internet, and landline phones were our means of communication. She was not in my house long until we were making love in my bed. I did not want to rush her, but in her eyes and touch; she told me she was ready. I had found another woman to fire my passion. Just how much her passion would rise meet mine, I did not yet know.

One thing led to another, and I invited her to live with me. After brief thought, she agreed, and moved in with me in Nyack. Here I was, living a dream of being a faculty at Cornell Medical College, and working towards my next dream of becoming a husband and father. Just how that happened, is a story in itself. I don't recall discussing when we would have children, only that we would. I am relatively certain she said she was not ready.

I also started seeing her moods. She would stay in her room for days, brood, angry, irritable, and depressed. I approached her in the same way I would with my patients. After all, she wanted to find a cure for her bulimic addiction, but not so much her moods. I reasoned with her that because I was in recovery from addictions, so could she be, with my help. You have to remember I was on a mission from God, and no challenge was too great. I faced my addictions in recovery, overcame my fears, moved to New York, and traveled alone throughout Europe. I thought I could handle a case of bulimia and dark moods. I was determined to fix her and have my family.

We had unprotected sex in my mind with the purpose of getting her pregnant to have children. I felt naturally compelled. Until this point in my life I had not impregnated anyone to my knowledge, after many sexual encounters. In our case, she became pregnant within weeks of her arrival with our first daughter. I was thrilled and she was pleased, but overwhelmed just the same. I had prepared for this moment for a long time, whereas she had not. Not long after she became pregnant, we were married in a Methodist Church. I had relatives from the New York area at the wedding, and we were married in Nyack as befitting our humble beginnings.

I had also lived with a woman and had been married once before so I knew what to expect. But she was different from the others. When she had her mood attacks, she would stay in her room for a day or so, have a disgusted look on her face. She was so angry. I approached her as I would a patient, and not necessarily as a sympathetic husband. I showed little tolerance for her behavior, and confronted her about these spells. She explained her father had similar episodes, and would break up the house, destroy furniture, and spew in rage at their family.

She called them moods, and I called them explosive attacks. A psychiatrist she saw diagnosed her as having Explosive Disorder. I was never seriously threatened physically by her, though she did make some physical attacks towards me. You have to remember I was invincible, on a mission, and had the shield of God in everything I did. I had survived a fatal overdose, jails, many years of dangerous intoxication, and who knows how many encounters with death. I had a purpose, had survived for a reason, and my relationship with my new wife I determined, was another challenge.

I had reduced my AA meeting attendance to once a week. I found a medium size meeting in a small river town on the Hudson in a colonial looking church, typical of the area. I led the meeting for a prolonged period of time, favoring my practice to serve and do a commitment as part of my recovery. My wife was not particularly fond of my outside interest in meetings. I felt she was controlling me. Sometimes I felt like I was engulfed by an octopus, being blocked from relationships with others. I am by nature a loner, so to not have abundant social contact was not an inconvenience, but her need to possess frustrated me.

Her pregnancy progressed, and the time came for her to deliver. Once again, I seemed to be ready, but she did not. We entered the birthing room sometime during the day. She was already having considerable pain from her uterine contractions. I was present in the room with her throughout the delivery, and exercised my medical, fatherly, and spousal judgment. She had a rather narrow birth canal, so she struggled during labor. After not too long the doctor informed us that the umbilical cord was wrapped around the fetus' neck, and was causing the pulse to slow, and some fetal distress.

The doctor wanted to perform a Cesarean Section as the mother was complaining of considerable pain, her pelvis aperture was tight, and the slow fetal heartbeat was endangering her oxygenation. I was reluctant for her to have a Cesarean at such as young age and asked if she could try more time as the surgical team entered the birthing room. I didn't want a young woman to have her gut split open if I could help it. In my usual approach to obstacles, I forcefully yelled as loud as I could, "Push, push, push!" To this day she remembers my exhortations mixed with the supreme pain she experienced from her contractions and pelvis bone separating under the pressure from the fetus' head, forcing its way under and out of the "Triumphal Arch."

When she came out, the baby was flush with color, and moved briskly. She had the cutest handle bar pink cheeks, and slit blue eyes, starring pensively. Her mother was done suffering, and baby undisturbed by the whole event of fighting for her life.

We put her in the back seat of the car in a booster seat, wrapped in bundles of blankets on that frigid January afternoon, and drove a short distance to our home in Nyack. When I placed her in her crib, her tiny self appeared lost in the space. She was quiet most of the time until two am when I heard a faint cry from her room. Instinctively I picked her up and brought her to her mother who breast-fed her. I placed her back in her crib without hearing from her until later in the morning, around eight in the morning. She did that for a month, like clockwork, and I would always pick her up to bring her to her mother.

After that she slept through the night until she became a teenager, when she instead slept long into the afternoon. When she was able to walk at one year, she acted like a "snip," no other way to describe it. Little did I know she was to become a carbon copy of me and her mother, shadowing me, eventually passing me in achievements. However, for natural reasons I suppose, daughter and mother did not mix, and were like oil and water. Both irritated the other.

Diane and I continued to have unprotected sex— I still wanted more children. But she was noticeably upset when the pregnancy test turned positive in the kitchen of our house and on the grounds of New York Hospital. She became depressed almost instantly, which lasted through post-partum. She complained carrying the fetus was uncomfortable, and wanted to deliver as soon as possible. She asked if we could have sexual intercourse to trigger onset of labor, and it worked. Not long after, we were in the birthing room again, but this time labor went without incident and the baby came out looking healthy as ever, strong and vital. I remember examining her as she lie on the table, moving all four arms and legs, and expressing quiet satisfaction with her new life. Quite a proud Daddy, and an exhausted and relieved mother.

However, a storm was brewing. My wife remained depressed after giving birth. She had a 19-month old child, and was now saddled with a newborn. She started having thoughts to harm self and the newborn baby. I was not much help as I focused on my work, and didn't really understand why she wasn't more thrilled and euphoric about our two lovely daughters.

What I now understand is she was suffering from Post-Partum Depression, where mothers are quite severely depressed with strange thoughts about harming self and child. These illogical thoughts do not rise out of animosity or malice, rather an illness of the mind. Post-partum depression is fairly common, and is usually self-remitting over 3 to 6 months. Treatment with antidepressant medications and psychotherapy can help with the symptoms, and careful monitoring of the mother for her thoughts is indicated. I had an AA friend who comforted her, and communicated her status to me.

Here I was, a psychiatrist in a leading psychiatric hospital who was running away from a psychiatric problem in my wife. I suppose I was handling her depression as I would my addiction, though she did not have the tools or support I did. She also was talking strangely to friends she had made on the grounds of the hospital. She did not talk to me about her feelings or thoughts. I just kept expecting her to pull herself together, and enjoy motherhood, husband, and family. But she did not seem to care about her daughters, or me. Her anger spurned my affection, and made it difficult for me to feel safe and secure around her.

I felt she was immature, but she was 19 years younger after all, and I possessed much more living and learning. She had not yet attended college, had no career. She had been raised in a troubled home life, carrying around genetic emotional turbulence. I was educated, in recovery, with an established career. But I was similar to her in a way. I didn't have a firm, stable emotional life either. I too was prone to emotional sensitivity, being highly reactive, with limited empathy. I carried an intolerant attitude towards weakness and became defensive when she emotionally and physically attacked. I provided whatever limited support as much as I could. She did not harm anyone, and gradually developed more self-control.

My career was progressing at the New York Hospital, Cornell Medical Center. We published a book on addictions that I had edited, which won a national award. I was publishing regularly with my famous colleague. We were on the national stage, and I was an Ivy Leaguer, married, and with beautiful children. I completely changed the Alcohol Treatment Unit from a Psychiatric perspective to an Addiction Perspective. It was a matter of focusing on addiction as an independent disease, as opposed to having a psychiatric disorder that caused addictive use of drugs and alcohol.

The aim was diagnosis and treatment of addictive disorders as primary, without being caused by underlying psychiatric disorder, and the specific addiction treatment to stop and prevent the preoccupation with acquiring alcohol and drugs, compulsive use or use despite adverse consequences, and relapse to alcohol and drugs. We detoxified individuals from alcohol and drugs, as we provided them education and group therapies, AA and Narcotics Anonymous (NA) meetings, and additional medical and psychiatric treatments as indicated. Most patients did not need additional psychiatric care, and many had tried psychiatric medications, psychotherapy, and other peripheral treatments without effect on their addictive drug use. Addicted patients needed to accept their addictive disease, and establish a commitment to recovery, usually in AA or NA. Not much progress could be made in their personality, mood, or interpersonal relationships if they continued to drink and use drugs.

My position was Unit Chief, responsible for the entire unit. I was able to set the treatment modes, supervise other physicians, residents, nurses, and therapists. The Alcohol and Drug Unit was a primary teaching site for addictions at Cornell University Medical College. On the Unit I trained Cornell Residents and Medical Students in Addiction Psychiatry with generally good satisfaction scores, and had trainees to go on and specialize in Addiction Psychiatry.

However, true to myself, and my intolerant approach I thought necessary for addiction treatment and recovery, I surrendered myself. In a meeting with my supervisors and administrators, I was instructed to change my Addiction Unit to a Dual Diagnosis Unit. I was not asked my thoughts, opinions, or experience in addiction treatment. I was not told who made the decision. I was not told I couldn't lead the new Dual Diagnosis Unit. My knee jerk response was, "You can find someone else to lead it." I would not compromise my focus on addictions because it worked, and the psychiatric approach did not.

Besides, I had been thinking about changing my career direction from a psychiatric based hospital to a more medical setting. I also wanted to return to the Midwest to be closer to my mother and the children's grandmother in Michigan. I had been ruminating about settling my family in more familiar surroundings, and exposing my daughters to their family heritage. I probably made the decision to make such a change when I returned their ultimatum with my ultimatum. Not long after my fateful declaration, I was informed my contract would not be renewed, and had a year before I had to leave. I suspected the Chair of the Department of Psychiatry made the decision to convert to a Dual Diagnosis Unit.

As planned, unconsciously and under the direction of the God of my Understanding, I interviewed for an opportunity at the University of Pennsylvania and the University of Illinois at Chicago. I was offered a job at Penn, but yielded to a return to my roots. So we packed up our belongings, and drove in our cars to the Chicago area. Where driving on the expressway was not necessary, but my wife still had access to city life.

I had a new start closer to my mother in Michigan,

and in a Department of Psychiatry at the University of Illinois at Chicago, headed by a long time Yale faculty member. I had landed on my feet in a major medical center and school. Many would consider it a promotion, at the rank of Associate Professor and Chief of Addiction Programs. My publications were booming, my national reputation as an author and clinician growing, and my credibility as an addiction expert launched.

But I still carried with me the same intransigent personality and unbending convictions and an attitude to be true to self. I would learn again the hard way there were looming consequences to my determined and uncompromising approach to my personal and professional lives. Unsuspectingly, I was about to experience another terrifying and challenging chapter to my life.

Well I've been waiting for this moment for all my life, oh Lord
I can feel it coming in the air tonight, oh Lord

—"In the Air Tonight" Phil Collins

12

POLITICS (Divorce And Termination)

*"I am seeking, I am striving, I am in it
with all my heart."* —Vincent Van Gogh

In my early days in sobriety, I used many simple but profound quotes that enlightened my understanding of my disease and recovery, and provided me with uncharacteristic clarity and profound peace. "First things first" reminded me to keep priorities in sobriety such as not taking that first drink, attending AA meetings, utilizing a sponsor, working and applying the steps to my life, and reading the Big Book of Alcoholics Anonymous. Further, "One drink is too many and a thousand are not enough," because of the loss of control over alcohol. My very favorite is, "Nothing is so bad that a drink won't make worse," meaning addictive drinking makes any problem unsolvable and more complicated, and increases my depression with a return of a feeling of hopelessness. Another favorite, "Let go, let God," is one I still use if I am tempted by or get an urge from alcohol. "Think, think, think a drink through," encourages me to remember where alcohol always took me in my darkest days of addiction. All these exhortations apply to the use of drugs similarly.

Can I stay sober and keep emotional balance under all conditions? And must I keep emotional balance to keep sober? Self-searching becomes a regular habit. My most important job is to stay away from the first drink or drug. Whether it makes sense or not, personal responsibility is key to avoid relapse. In doing so I keep my emotions under control, or at least from being out of control too far, by reflecting my role in conflict. What did I do to create a stir in myself or others? I must admit, accept, and patiently correct my defects or wrong actions. Bulldozing ahead will not lead to a resolution. I also learned that if I maintained self-control, I would be more apt to be successful and achieve my goals. As well as avoid emotional hangovers that just made everything worse. These tall tasks take me to Step 10: "Continued to take personal inventory and when we were wrong promptly admitted it."

After my past was settled with the previous steps, present challenges could be met without taking a drink or losing ground on my ambitions. There are varieties of inventories, instincts of anger, resentments, jealously, envy, self-pity, hurt, pride, all of which are common emotions that can lead to a relapse. Self-restraint, however, difficult to exert, and resist in place of justifiable anger, is my first objective. This step is insurance against "big-shot-ism" and grandiosity, which cloud my judgments and decisions. At the same time, this Step is an opportunity to assess credits as well as debits. I found that I could examine my motives and those of others.

Don't ask me why this self-appraisal is necessary to keep sober. I really don't know. I know that the center for addiction to drugs and alcohol in the brain is near the emotions. And possibly too high an emotional activity could trigger relapse to alcohol and drugs. After all, alcohol and drugs alter emotions, which is a main attraction to their use. Such as a light goes on, feelings of euphoria and well-being are present in the beginning, later replaced by a negative and hopeless state as the addictive drive takes over with the deepening addiction of alcohol and drugs.

It is a spiritual axiom that every time we are disturbed, no matter what the cause, there is something wrong *with us.* If somebody hurts us and we are sore, we are in the wrong also. You can ponder that axiom or just accept as I do, as hard to understand. I know it is a valuable axiom because it tells me to look at myself in all conditions, with everyone, at all times, if I want to truly know what happened, particularly with emotional reactions.

What does that have to do with my story? Well I became embroiled in an extremely contentious divorce proceeding with my wife, and mother of my two daughters. I was deeply captured in four years of continuous conflict and antagonism, in disagreements and arguments, principally, over custody of our children. The acrimony eventually led to unspeakable and catastrophic consequences from which we are still in recovery years later.

My feeling is that the current divorce practices according to laws and attorneys often do more harm than good, and have harmful outcomes for all concerned, except maybe the attorneys who collect money as a result of client grief and anger that prolongs the legal conflicts. I had to exercise a degree of self-restraint I never thought possible to avoid harm to my daughters.

You can imagine the anger and resentments constantly plaguing our struggle over custody. At one point in our proceedings, I was about to cave in to the stereotype and become the visitation father in spite of being the predominant parent up to that point. But my use of the 10th Step told me to hang in there for the best interest of the children, as I didn't think their mother had the maturity and means to raise them on her own. Our battle over custody lasted about four years, with very little progress until the very end. As is often the case, the contention did not end with the divorce. However, I later found out in a big way why she wanted permanent sole custody of both daughters.

I was hired to be the Addiction Specialist in Department of Psychiatry at University of Illinois in Chicago. I really wasn't thrilled about moving to Chicago from the Mecca and excitement in New York, and stepping down from the prestigious Ivy League Medical School. I had left a high profile position to assume Midwestern mediocrity. However, the new Chair was a longtime Yale professor, and I was recommended by Dr. Scott Kirby, a Yale graduate. Previously, I didn't want to work in a VA Hospital particularly because I wanted to provide addiction services to larger populations, and show the world that addictive diseases occurred outside troubled and poorly motivated veterans.

Guess what? I ended up taking a position at the University of Illinois at Chicago, spending some of my time at the Westside VA where I had spent a period of my residency in Internal Medicine. I was stuck in a building separated from the main hospital, seeing pretty severely affected, down and out alcoholics and drug addicted veterans.

I had angered the Chief of Psychiatry at the VAH, which came back big to haunt me. He didn't think I devoted enough attention to his conception of my duties. I do think he applied a higher standard to me. He didn't like the Chair at UIC, and therefore tortured me as an intermediary messenger. I was pretty miserable and a target for the political infighting, plenty of that at the VA and UIC. I am always reminded I was raised to be honest and hardworking, but the "P word" was not mentioned much; politics were pretty absent in my upbringing. It was so lacking, my parents wouldn't even tell me who they voted for and what political parties they identified with. I was just a Jewish Catholic from a divorced home, who was going to college someday, somewhere, to become a professional man. But I also could develop addiction programs for the main University Hospital, and teach programs in Addiction Psychiatry. Eventually I developed consultation programs in addictions in concert with medicine services. I supervised a detoxification program in the hospital, and outpatient addiction treatment services. Also, I developed a fellowship in Addiction Psychiatry and continued to publish medical journal articles and books in addictions. I became nationally known and regarded as an expert in my field. I wrote at a feverish pace, and advanced my mission in print form.

Miraculously, I was accomplishing what I set out to do in Minnesota by carrying a message to the world about addictions. I was rapidly learning that most people didn't want to know about addictions, and inexplicably got away with ignoring it to the detriment of those afflicted with addictions. Their motto was, "See no evil, hear no evil, speak no evil." The general public believed: addictions are evil, caused by evil, and cause evil, and were moral issues, not medical. To them it was like sex, not talked about, but frequently practiced.

I had a chairman who was supportive to a point. He also had grand scheme for the Department that did not include me. There was an heir apparent, Ross Doherty, who did not care for my defiant, joking attitude, and he was relatively ruthless. He had a reputation for female harassment, and other questionable personality traits, and was not popular among his peers. Nevertheless, he rose to the top of the political heap in the Department of Psychiatry and eventually the Medical School as Dean. He turned out to be my death knoll at UIC.

Upon arriving in Chicago, Diane, daughters, and I moved into an apartment on Lake Shore Drive. I passed up an opportunity to rent with option to buy in a suburb, Oak Park. I am not sure why I made the decision to live in the city, except I disdain commutes, particularly, in heavy traffic. The westbound expressway, the Eisenhower, is generally packed at rush hour, and I thought Diane could better adapt to city life. As it turned out, our lives may have taken a different course had we not settled in the city.

Our younger daughter, Anya walked for the first time in our living room after she crawled for a month or two. She was a sturdy young child from day one, hard to topple over. On the other hand, from a young age Kate was screaming when she was with her mother, they never got along together, like mixing oil and water. Not sure why except maybe they were so much alike. Both temperamental, trying to control anger underneath, fighting to hold in explosive outbursts, tense with measured emotional release.

Initially, I admit I did not assume much responsibility for the young children. Mother had an au pair to help her, and she did not work. She eventually started and finished college at the University of Illinois at Chicago in Art and Design. All while she and I gradually had withdrawn from each other. She had increasingly violent outbursts and attacked me verbally and physically on a regular basis. I could not handle her explosive attacks frequently focused on me, as I did not see it anywhere else from anyone else. I am pretty reactive myself emotionally.

Though I knew she was disturbed, I could not restrain myself from reacting to her overpowering anger. We saw a counselor but I had trouble with his lack of focus on her behaviors, whatever our problems might have been. He kept analyzing her difficulties, while not instructing her to stop or control her attacks on me.

I did not strike out at her, and I may have upset her at times, but her attacks were out of proportion to my acts and behaviors, in my estimation. I wonder how anyone would hold up after repeated attacks with verbal accusations and having objects thrown at you, objects broken, constant criticisms, and trying to control another's life. I had few friends, did not do many activities outside her reach, and did not play much of a role in the children's care. I eventually refused to have sex with her as I saw her as furious, petulant child, which enraged her even more, and caused me to recoil, to intensify my defenses. I did not have an adult relationship with her, emotionally or physically. I could see maybe why she sought intimacy with someone else but I was constantly deflecting and retreating from her anger.

While at a conference, I called one night from out of town and she did not answer. That was unusual and I suspected something then. She indeed had initiated an affair with another man, who I later found out was a Peruvian diplomat stationed in Chicago. I knew at this point we were headed for separation, infidelity. I had never been unfaithful to her, though I had opportunities. I had decided I simply could not live with the anger and attacks. She had decided she could not live with my provocations, according to her. We accused each other of over controlling. And now, finally, she had found another man.

She filed for a divorce with a mediating attorney and moved out of the apartment. A sinking, empty feeling overcame me. But I looked forward to peace from the turmoil and conflict. She agreed to leave the kids with me four days per week, and alternating weekends. She found an apartment in Lincoln Park, not far from me. She had not definitively decided to divorce me and looked for mediation. I had decided I didn't want to go back to the fighting.

Without any prior training, I just naturally started caring for the girls, ages 2 and nearly 4 years old. Don't ask me how I did it. I was working full-time at the Medical Center. I hired an au pair to begin with, and eventually had childcare during the day when the girls were not in preschool. From the start, I taught them to care for themselves, pick out their clothes, bathe themselves, and entertain and occupy their time. I took them for walks, regular stints in the parks. I suddenly became a mother and father. With sadness, I remember taking each of them by their hands and walking down Michigan Avenue to the FAO Schwartz toy store and Watertower to look around, and shop. A favorite stop was a candy store where we loaded up.

Eventually, we moved from the apartment to a condominium I purchased a few blocks away. The girls seemed comfortable going back and forth to my place and their mother's. They were enrolled in a private school of Diane's choice at the beginning based on her European education. I had a sitter for afterschool that the mother openly objected to. Our agreed upon custody routine, four days with me and three days with their mother worked, up to a point. But we continued to argue over choice of school, after school activities, sports, religion, and extracurricular activities. We alternated weekends, holidays, and vacations in the typical custody agreements. I took the girls to Michigan to visit my mother. They established a relationship with their grandmother from an early age, and she also visited us in Chicago.

The girls and I joined an Episcopal Church and they attended Sunday School. I became a member and usher, and we participated in the church life, which later was a great source of power and support. To begin with, their mother objected to early religious education, and expressed displeasure with their baptism, and later confirmation, though she did attend the events. A particularly fun and meaningful time was Christmas when the kids participated in the Christmas Pageants, one was a sheep and the other a shepherd. I had found a family in the Church, and I looked forward to Sundays.

I prayed harder and harder, and didn't know I was preparing for the biggest blow of my life second to the alcoholism and drug addiction. I had always tried to follow the suggested list of priorities in order, sobriety in AA, family, career. Having children and being a predominant parent was still second to staying sober and practicing the steps in AA. Knowing, without AA, it would all fall apart.

I continued to attend AA meetings held in the same church, meet with my sponsor, and work the steps. Diane challenged me to work the 10th Step, as my emotional balance was definitely stretched by our persistent disagreements over how to raise the girls. I did not react to her negative attacks on me, nor her basic conflicts over just about everything, from how to dress the girls to school, to my having childcare instead of her (even though she had started to work and used childcare herself).

She had hired a new attorney and I hired one as well, and that's when all hell broke loose. To me, her new attorney was like her, a bulldog, demanding, dogmatic, and wanted the whole pie, permanent sole custody. I could not bring myself to agree to turn raising the girls over to the mother. She was too unstable and volatile. And she was foreign with citizenship in Switzerland and Germany, not the United States. I foresaw in the future she would try to take them to a foreign country, and would do so easier if she had sole custody.

We continued a four-year contentious and brutal battle over custody of the children. I moved the girls from the mother's school to a private school close to our condo. However, I couldn't enroll the girls in activities with our divided schedules, and so the girls could not play soccer or attend other afterschool activities. And she continued to demand permanent, sole custody of the children. I never completely understood why until later.

I recall a day when I wanted to give in to her demands for custody and could see why men caved in to such pressures. But I just followed the legal standard of the "*best interest of the child*," in this case as the father, and continued to fight for custody. I also did not want the kids to be stretched between two homes, especially one side that could not financially and emotionally care for the children. I naturally wanted to make a home for them.

Initially, Diane and I were ordered to have an evaluation for custody by a social worker, who initially sided with Diane as the mother and recommended physical custody to her. I think the girls understood that they could lose a parent, particularly, their mother, and were intimidated by the process.

Finally however, the children's attorney sided with me for sole custody. She made her decision based on my actions to help Anya get surgery for her tonsils. Anya had stopped breathing at night because of obstruction from her enlarged tonsils. Diane opposed the surgery on philosophical grounds, not medical. To settle the matter in Anya's interest, I accepted Diane's proposal to let Anya stay with her post operatively if she agreed to surgery. The attorney thought I was acting in the child's best interest and not mine, and Diane was doing the opposite by opposing surgery, then agreeing to it if she could have the child with her after surgery.

Surprisingly, the girls seemed to do well, and weather the storm around them from us. I did not do as well and became so depressed that my boss had me evaluated by another psychiatric faculty member because of my seriously sad state. I then realized the toll the separation and strife and parenting had on my psychic well-being. Diane by then was in a relationship with the man she had had the affair with. The girls saw him but I had never met him.

In the meantime, I developed an approved fellowship in Addiction Psychiatry, Addiction Detoxification Service in the UIC Hospital, teaching programs for Medical Students and Residents, joined the Liver Transplantation Team, obtained membership in College Curriculum Committee, continued The Medical Education Committee, and published many articles and books. In spite of my achievements, I was given notice that my contract at UIC was not going to be renewed. Added as a contrived justification was that I was also accused of sexual harassment during my review for tenure and promotion.

I believed the inquisition was orchestrated by Dr. Ross Doherty, the Heir Apparent to the Chair to the Department of Psychiatry. In response, I sued the medical school, Doherty and Alan Staughan. As a settlement I was given a year's salary and time off. It came at a very opportune time as I later found out.

Things went from bad to worse. The next chapter of my life was not a surprise, but still a shock and not anticipated in its entirety. My lawyer did not see it coming, and completely dropped the ball. I began to understand Diane's determination to get custody. and it was not only for possessiveness and domination. She had anger and frustration, and other ideas in mind, not in the best interest of the children, and certainly not me. The standard I had to meet to obtain custody of the girls was the "best interest" of the children, balanced against the rights of the parents was a legal decision ultimately.

According to my attorney at the time, the best interest of the child boiled down to the parent who could provide the most stable physical and emotional environment and security, not necessarily the parent who could provide the best economic support. Though I did not see how economic support wasn't in the best interest of the child as well.

Mothers, of course, are favored, due to their perceived supportive emotional nature, and nurturing feminine qualities, just being the mothers. I considered Diane's emotional nature too unstable and volatile for the best interest of our daughters. While the direct economic support was not a heavily weighed factor in the best interest standard, I included it in my decision-making. I wanted the girls to have the better things, such as good health and education, family environment, and security. Diane was foreign and involved with a foreign diplomat. I could easily see her taking the kids to another country apart from me and my family.

She certainly showed no signs of being able to support the children financially. Her rages and anger towards me spelled her desire to separate the children from me. She always thought I was trying to keep her separated from the children. Not true, but I did think some structure and a home for the children was important. And I was the most likely to be able to provide that continuity and stability.

I always thought the possibility of harm from Diane's explosiveness and anger outweighed other factors. I certainly cared about safety concerns, given her physical attacks on me. The care, protection, and safety of the children's well being were paramount to me. I fought for their survival and development, generally ensured best by remaining in or maintaining close contacts with the family and their social and cultural networks. Not possible if Diane took them to Germany or another foreign country. Her focus was on her own life, and what possibilities lay ahead for her. She was not focused on the children's family and social life in the U.S., with my family and relatives.

My practice of Step 10 was to minimize as much as possible my contributions to the conflicts. What could I do to monitor my resentments, anger, and self-centered fear to avoid losing ground in my battle for custody? I certainly feared Diane and her emotional outbursts. How could she rear the children with her moods? Would she take the children to a foreign country and eliminate me from their lives? I became very resentful towards her blocking my attempts for the children to play soccer, attend traditional schools, to have a nice place to live and not her one-bedroom apartment, to provide economic advantages. How could I avoid showing anger to her accusations, allegations, and demeaning voice? How could I separate my selfish desire to raise my children my way and not divide them into halves? How could I talk to Diane when she didn't want to talk with me? How could I refrain from retaliation to all these intense emotional, acrimonious battles?

What I learned from the contentious divorce, particularly over custody proceedings, was that the current adverse legal structure for divorce acts to make all these negative emotions worse, and to intensify barriers to communications. Not to mention, the protracted course that places lives and decisions on hold, e.g. school, home environment, and expensive legal bills. In my case the impending doom of the unknown fate of my children, in some distant land, with someone whose actions caused me to fear for their safety.

Our divorce proceedings took four years, and may have ended sooner if Diane did not have other plans. My attorney calculated that I was an older man, and the children were girls, and seemed more concerned about my anger in court despite the assigned girls' attorney approval of me. In those four years, I became depressed, worried, emotionally drained, embattled, and distraught. I had to fight for normalcy for the children, such as religious training, baptism, confirmation, schools, dress, without any credit for a job well done.

At one point, Diane had recorded a conversation where I had raised my voice in frustration and anger after she deliberately provoked me. The attorney thought I would lose in a trial in court if the recording was played in court. It would confirm Diane's accusations that I was the male stereotype: controlling, bullying, insensitive, angry, unreasonable, unfit father.

After the girls' attorney declared it was in the girls' best interest for me to be the custodial parent, the bitter battle over custody finally ended in November 1997, after four years of contentious acrimony. Diane and I agreed to joint legal custody and my physical custody, which meant I was the custodial parent. The schedule and school for the children remained the same, per my choice.

I also learned through these legal proceedings that the court does not like to change prior joint agreements without compelling reasons, and here there was none. Although I had expressed worry about Diane's planned trip to Germany to visit her parents, I was told by my attorney I could do nothing prevent it. I asked my attorney Debbie

Jones to block the trip for now. She refused based on her opinion I could not prevent Diane's planned trip; a mistake with grave consequences and lasting repercussions. I delayed an opportunity to sue for legal malpractice to recoup my upcoming expenses. However, the attorney was instrumental later in preserving my custody rights.

I vividly remember Diane telling the girls to say goodbye to me on the steps of my condominium as they left on her vacation to Germany in July 1997. While I didn't know exactly the plans Diane had in mind, I had a sinking sense that she would try something. I continued to beg the attorney to stop her. I did not know for just how long at that time their vacation would last. My surprise was where the vacation would take place, and with whom. And that I was soon to be out of a job, unemployed. Diane told the girls to give me a "big hug." So they did. They didn't know either how our lives would be changed forever. No job, kids or wife. Running on empty, but with hope and direction.

And you coming back to me is against the odds
And that's what I've got to face

—"Against All Odds" Phil Collins

13

ABDUCTION

"Many stokes, though with little axe,
hew down and fell the hardest-timber'd oak."
—William Shakespeare

"**P**lease check whether my daughters are on the flight from Frankfort to Chicago for today," I asked the clerk at the American Airlines Counter in Chicago. "I'm not supposed to tell you, but I do not find that your daughters are on board that plane, their seats are empty." I had no further answer when I called for the children in Kassel, Germany. I had previously been able to speak with them on a regular basis during their stay. It was unusual for no one to answer at her parents' home where Diane and the daughters were staying. So, I became worried and decided to go to the Airline to confirm if my daughters were indeed on the flight.

It was then I was confronted with a mystery and my worst fears. Where were the girls and Diane? I waited until their arrival time at O'Hara Airport. No word from them. I knew there was trouble but did not know the extent. I couldn't think that far ahead. This had never happened to me before.

I finally got Diane's father on the telephone. In his heavy German accent, he answered "Northern Germany," when I asked where the girls and Diane were. Otherwise, he was not willing to say anything more and hung up. He sounded far, far away. I felt my daughters were far, far away and I had no plan at that time. I had never been in such a predicament in my life. I remember losing a puppy as a child and searching for it for days on my bicycle. Believe it or not I found it wandering one day, and brought it home. Now here I was again, looking for lost puppies, my eight and nine year-old daughters.

Soon after, I met with my attorney who drew up a motion for the court. On the wall in the courtroom, hung a sign inscribed, "In God We Trust." I started with God there and found out about the power of the law and God, as I searched for them. The judge issued an order to hold Diane in contempt of court and awarded me "sole permanent custody" of my daughters, leaving Diane with no legal rights to the children. But I did not have them.

My next step was to take the court order to a Chicago Police station to obtain an arrest warrant for Diane. As I walked into the police station, a male police officer laughed at me when I said my children were kidnapped, "Oh sure buddy, and what do you want me to do about it?" Not an auspicious beginning.

A female police officer overhead us, and sat me down at a desk and filled out a report and warrant for the arrest of Diane for Child Abduction. She was sympathetic and supportive. I was angered over the other officer's rude thoughtlessness, so typical of Chicago police officers, so macho and demeaning. And the female officer immediately brought hope to me.

Eventually I turned the Chicago arrest warrant into a national warrant, LEEDS, and registered within the United States. According to the LEEDS, Diane would be arrested if she tried to pass through U.S. immigrations. But it did not extend to foreign countries. I now held a document I could take to the world and eventually international courts, governments, consulates, ambassadors, congressman, U.S. Senators, Immigration, private detectives, police and to anyone who would listen and could help me find and return my daughters.

I checked out Diane's apartment in Lincoln Park. It was empty. No sign of her or children. She had left the Honda Accord I had bought her in my condominium garage. I had only memories of the children and emotional scars from my battles with Diane. Still a hopeful attitude persisted in me. I did not, could not, think how life would be without the girls. I continued one day at a time, adding people who could help anywhere in the world. My search was becoming truly international. I had no boundaries to my search, heaven and earth.

My attorney suggested I go to Germany. I found an AA friend who spoke fluent German to accompany me to Kassel, and we left almost immediately on the plane. We arrived to check into a Ramada Hotel. Right away, I headed to the grandparents house, and met with her father. He again told me that they went to Northern Germany for a Holiday, and he didn't know when they would return. As I pressed him for more information, and hoping against hope that the girls were with them in the house, he threatened to call the police.

Imagine that, he helped steal my children, and he was going to have me arrested. I didn't want to end up in a German jail. I wanted to continue to search for the girls and couldn't do it incarcerated. I was already beginning to realize I had to stay healthy and free. I had to exercise caution to save myself and the girls.

Sometime after my arrival, I received a call from my

attorney who suspected Diane and the girls went to Peru, in South America to live with her boyfriend, Luis. She had gone to the Peruvian Consult in Chicago and spoke with Luis who denied everything. At that point, I had no further business in Kassel, and left to return to the U.S. Before leaving I was beginning to learn about the power of the law when I took my documents to courts in Germany. My court order, awarding me sole custody, LEEDS arrest warrant, and identification as an American doctor attracted attention and credibility, or at least acknowledgment. Now however, I was really beginning to worry, my girls in South America? It was then, a wave of hopelessness hit me. It was then I began thinking I would never see them again.

I found myself turning to an unlikely character from the past, Jesus Christ. Despite previously causing me great conflict with my Jewish beliefs, I decided to go to Saint Chrysostums church and meet with the Minister. He announced the abduction in Church and asked for the parishioners' prayers. As a Jew, I prayed to Christ at the Crucifixation Cross to help me to return my daughters. In return, I would be obligated to Him.

I had previously been able to attend the Episcopal Church without worrying too much about Christ. Just seeking a spiritual connection, and communication with a power greater than myself, and I accepted at least that. I looked for that power in many places. But I had wanted my children to have a religious experience, and Diane would never approve of a Catholic Church. She really didn't approve of any formal religion, which was yet another conflict. But there I was, looking for help anywhere and from anyone to get my daughters back. Even if it meant teaming up with Jesus Christ himself, hooray.

I remember in the church, there was a large statute

of Christ on the altar. I looked at it every time I was there searching for more power, and to improve my conscious contact with a power greater than myself.

I took on Step 11 for direction and power in my search for my daughters: *"Sought through prayer and meditation to improve our conscious contact with God as we understood Him, praying only for knowledge of His will for us and the power to carry that out."*

Prayer and meditation are my principle means of conscious contact with God, in my case my Higher Power. I started acting as if meditation and prayer were my main channels to my Higher Power, mostly through actions. The hard part was establishing a connection between self-examination and meditation and prayer. I had already learned that these actions were an unshakable foundation for life. How shall I meditate? Meditation has no boundaries, and South America was a long way away. I initiated an individual adventure to many places and with many people, one step and one day at a time.

The first result of meditation is emotional balance. Above all I needed emotional balance to pursue and convince others to help me return my daughters. I knew that crying, screaming, and jumping up and down was not going to get me very far. I remained conscious that I was the father, and the mother abducted the children. The natural inclination was to think I had done something to make the mother to take them from me, like domestic or child abuse. I had to keep my senses about me at all times; my daughters' lives were at stake. No time for self-righteous indignation or petty resentments to block my mission to return my daughters.

What about prayer? My prayers were daily petitions for understanding of God's will and the grace to carry it out. In this case, to return my daughters. The actual results of prayer are beyond question. Rewards of meditation and prayer are immeasurable. The tricky part was to search for God's will, not mine, as I could not expect according to Step 11, to specifically take this troubling dilemma to God, and secure from Him definite answers to my requests to return my daughters. Although I did ask Jesus Christ to help me, imagine that. However, I was determined to secure guidance and uncover new resources of courage. I increasingly discovered a sense of belonging with the members of the Church, my family, and having purpose to my mission rather than a frightened, grief stricken, reckless, purposeless search. While trite, I discovered in my prayer and meditation that God does move in mysterious ways, His wonders to perform. Really, He did for me.

I practiced meditation and prayer on the go, and I thought throughout the day. I was never good just sitting and pondering truth and God's will. Rather, I had to act it out and find answers in taking actions. Prayer to me was another action. I still used my conception of the unmoved mover, and I had to connect to be moved in a direction towards God's will. To me that meant the most successful solution to a problem, and life can be a problem to solve. I had problems the size of the world. I had to search from here to kingdom come. I had "willed" to bring my daughters into the world, now had to "will" to bring them back into my world.

This time I would try to do God's will, not mine, as before. My prayers were directed towards a power greater than myself. I had to admit I could not find and return them by myself. I had to rely on an unmoved mover to motivate and sustain my efforts, to keep hope, to overcome insurmountable odds. To me, South America was the end of the world.

Child abduction or theft is the unauthorized removal of a minor from their legally appointed guardians. Parental child abduction is the most common kind (200,000 domestically in 2010 alone), and is when a *parent* with unauthorized custody removes the child without mutual parental agreement or legal ruling. As you can imagine, this often occurs around parental separation/divorce, when one parent is assuming an advantage or is maybe afraid of losing the child in custody proceedings. But it also occurs in cases of alienation or abuse. A parent may refuse to return a child or flee with them in fear if domestic abuse is taking place. My resistance in the continuous custody battle was I had feared child abuse by Diane.

Child abduction can happen as close as the same city or state, or can span across nations or continents. International parental child abduction is when the child is taken out of country in violation of a custody or visitation agreement. Or, like in my situation, where the children are taken on an alleged vacation to a foreign country and are not returned. International cases are particularly difficult to resolve due to the conflicting international jurisdictions and laws, and the possible looming criminal prosecution or deportation charges the abducting parent could face in the child's home country, should they return.

The Hague Convention on the Civil Aspects of International Child Abduction is a multilateral human rights treaty designed to ensure the return of children abducted by a parent, back to the country of their habitual residence. Unfortunately, the treaty doesn't relieve most cases, so private parties are often hired by families, as I did.

Soon after finding out Diane had abducted the children with Luis Fernandez her Peruvian boyfriend, I met with his superior, the Chief Consulate in the Peruvian Embassy in Chicago. He was a gentlemanly man who listened to me patiently and empathetically. I explained my disheartening loss, and desire to return my daughters to their only and natural home, and how I believed his employee, Luis, abducted them with their mother, Diane. I had lodged my protest as I would to anyone who would listen. While he claimed he did not know anything about it, he promised to investigate back in Lima, Peru where Luis had been reassigned. I had another flicker of hope; my request had been accepted.

When I left, I began to realize I could put pressure on Luis and Diane from a distance through others closer than me. Being a father in a custody battle, particularly international, was a distinct disadvantage, as mothers are favored as always right. But my focus on the law and determined pleas for the safe return of my daughters from foreign lands to their home in the U.S. was God's will for me. I was the most political I have ever been in my life, even to this day. Remember, my dilemma was a lack of power.

My attorney advised me to get a private detective to help me locate and retrieve the girls. We knew that these high profile types worked inside and outside the law, and maneuvered with and without traditional law enforcement assistance. Media reports of private detectives re-abducting children back to their country of origin were well known. We had such a celebrity in Chicago, Ernie Rizzo, a wily, pugnacious private detective who worked on a dizzying array of high-profile cases, enough to keep tabloids both newsprint and video in material for years.

Among the many cases he claimed were assembling evidence of child abuse against Michael Jackson, searching for Paula Jones' father on behalf of President Clinton, and examining voice evidence against Mr. Clinton on behalf of CBS when the president denied having, "Sexual relations with that woman." Other files in his cabinet included work for or against Michael Jordan, Rep. Henry Hyde, William Kennedy Smith, O.J. Simpson, and Elian Gonzalez, the involuntary Cuban immigrant whom Rizzo planned to abduct and return to his father in Cuba, the detective told the New York Post. Using an array of high-tech, brains, and chutzpah, he always got his man. Or at least that was how he portrayed himself in a seemingly endless string of appearances on television and in print.

I never actually met Ernie, only talked with him on the phone. My attorney introduced me to him. We gave him vital information regarding my daughters, such as copies of birth certificates, photos, descriptions, and other personal data. And of course, I wired him $10,000 on initiation of work. He proved to be very useful. He and a partner flew to Lima, Peru, where he found an exceptional piece of information: an immigration record of Diane, Kate, and Anya leaving Lima, and traveling to Quito, Ecuado, with no intention of return. Now I knew at least where they probably were, but did not know why.

Diane had become a fugitive in deep parts of South America. I was living a nightmare. This was not according to my plan. How could I protect them thousands of miles away, in hostile lands? Would I ever see them again? Ernie didn't feel safe in Lima for long, that didn't help. He didn't want to go to Quito to find the girls. He ended his job with me. But I had the immigration record. I had the next step in my search.

I then tried to go to the FBI. They didn't want any involvement in the abduction. Child abduction was not something they wanted to do. I left the FBI office in Chicago empty handed. Somehow, I reasoned that I might be able to use political and government power to influence the Peruvian Consulate to pressure Luis. After all this was an international affair. So I met with then Senator Carol Mosely Braun, an African American woman who represented Illinois in the U.S. Senate. I spoke with a staff member who took my information.

Do you know what? Senator Mosely Braun came through for us. She wrote a letter with a copy to me to the Peruvian Ambassador in Washington D.C. In the letter, Senator Mosely Braun asked him to investigate my allegations of child abduction by one of his diplomats. My next step was to actually visit the Ambassador in Washington D.C., which I did. I met with two assistants who spent my time denying that Luis would do such a thing but agreed to investigate further. I sensed I was making progress by applying politic and diplomatic pressure through high levels.

I think the pressure I put on Luis and Diane caused her to flee from Lima to Quito. She became a fugitive from the law, another mistake on her part. I don't think Luis liked the questions posed to him by his consulate at work. He certainly did not want to answer to my allegations of child abduction, which could have been an international scandal, I suppose. I had convinced him and Diane with my arrest warrant that that she could face charges in the U.S., and I might be able to petition for her extradition. I also filed and served a civil law suit for child abduction to both Diane and Luis in Peru, demanding a million dollars. Next, I had two U.S. Senators, as I also enjoined the other Senator from Illinois, Dick Durbin, to support my pleas, as well as a U.S. Congressman, internationally known private detectives, and the U.S. State Department inquiring about the whereabouts of my children.

I met with U.S. Congressman Rod Blagojevich, who was enthusiastic about helping me return my daughters to the United States. He later became notorious as the 40th Governor of Illinois who accepted solicited bribes for political appointments. Once exposed, he was ultimately impeached, convicted, and sentenced to 14 years in federal prison for it. Though he later went on to become a convicted felon, in our interactions he was a decent, devoted father himself, who believed in helping me and my daughters.

I traveled to the U.S. State Department in Washington D.C. at the same time I paid a visit to complain to the Peruvian Ambassador. I met with staff workers in the State Department who explained the Hague Convention to me and assisted in my application. It all sounded good, except that the member country had to agree to assist a foreign plaintiff against a citizen of their own country. Diane was a German citizen, so I would have an uphill battle if she returned to Germany to fight my custody of the children. Likewise, I would have had a battle in Peru and Ecuador if I tried to go through courts. Moreover, Ecuador, not Peru, was a member of the Hague Convention.

Luckily, Diane and Luis chose to not defend against me in a Peruvian court. If they had done so, I could still be litigating a long drawn out case in court over custody. Diane instead chose to remain an illegal fugitive in a South American country where police and immigration officials are routinely bribed to capriciously enforce the law. That practice could become paramount in my attempts to return my daughters home. I could circumvent the red tape around immigrations with money.

A word about the power of the law. Wherever I went I showed the Court Order from the Chicago Probate Court that awarded me permanent sole custody of the girls and held Diane in contempt of court, along with the LEEDS for the arrest of Diane for Child Abduction. Courts in Germany, Switzerland, and governments in Peru and Ecuador, assisted me in my efforts to find and return my daughters based strongly on that as supported by other documentation. The power of the law reached thousands of miles, and influenced and persuaded countries and countless ordinary folks. I had Chicago police officers now assisting me in communicating with foreign police. I had the U.S. government, Senators, Congressmen, and foreign Consulates and Embassies, Immigration Police acknowledge my pleas on behalf of my daughters and executing official acts to assist a father and U.S. citizen.

Overseeing all these influential characters was the God of my Understanding. I maintained conscious contact with that power, as I did not have the power sufficient on my own to work with these officials and countries. I did not have the power to sustain my efforts despite being thousands of miles away and unable to see or touch people and places. My prayer and meditation were daily. I wish I could say that I prayed *only* for knowledge of His will for me and the power to carry it out, but I didn't. I prayed for the power to return my daughters, and all the people, governments, and countries to work with me.

Fortunately, I didn't expect and demand results overnight, and gradually began to see that I accomplished movements towards my goal. I had located Diane and the children in Quito. I had isolated and muted Luis's influence in Lima. I had gained the confidence of Senators, Congressman, U.S. State Department through my conscious contact with a higher power.

I was still attending AA meetings, working the other

Steps of AA to maintain my sobriety. I had not let up on my desire not to drink or use drugs. If anything, I realized more that I could not possibly carry out my quest drunk and drugged. I was searching against enough odds, as only a minority of parents successfully retrieve their abducted children. Yet I did not lose hope, and my determination grew. At this point in time I had lost my job, lost my children, but not my resolve.

I had to invade Quito, locate Diane and daughters, and swoop down and physically regain custody. I needed the next step. I found that step in the private detective, Anthony Pellicano. He had the experience, knowhow and power I lacked; he was the missing link between the law and justice. The grey areas where he operated were holes in the international laws to return children. He could unite the characters involved, and execute the Court Order from the Chicago Probate Court. He was God's will for me.

Workin' on a mystery, goin' wherever it leads
I'm runnin' down a dream

—"Runnin' Down a Dream" Tom Petty

14

HOPE (Return Of Children)

*"Hope is itself a species of happiness, and, perhaps,
the chief happiness which the world affords."*
—Samuel Johnson

I soon realized that my lost job provided time to make daily inquiries and travel around the world. A day at a time I made a call or took some step that moved me closer to my goal to retrieve my girls. I recall watching, in the meantime, the University of Michigan win the National Championship in 1997. I took solace in the familiar. My mother and sister were at my side. Nobody blamed me for anything. I didn't spend much time either blaming Diane, my focus was on returning the girls to me. When meeting with others, I gained much more attention and support by explaining my position and history with my daughters than rekindling arguments between Diane and me. I avoided re-creating drama around a dysfunctional relationship and who was right or wrong. I began with the power of the law and advanced my court order, awarding me sole custody and holding her in contempt of court. And an arrest warrant for Diane for child abduction.

I had to carefully assess my emotional balance to keep on an even keel and beam to maintain my effectiveness. I could not afford to wallow in self-pity, anger, resentments, or self-centered acts. I utilized Step 10 to control and avoid depression and feelings of hopelessness over the magnitude of my tasks. I carefully sidestepped conflicts, blaming, and regrets to maintain my momentum to move forward, closer to my daughter. Step 10, "Continued to take personal inventory and when we were wrong promptly admitted it." In working this step, I was able to recruit help from expected and unexpected sources. I maintained credibility and garnered support

My attorney, Debbie, was the one who put me in touch with Anthony Pellicano, a high profile Hollywood private investigator, whose client list included Michael Jackson, Farrah Fawcett, Chris Rock, and Arnold Schwarzenegger, to name a few. Pellicano was an early adapter of audio surveillance. Which, a decade later, would cost him 15 years in federal prison for "conspiracy to commit wiretapping," among other things. At the time I met him however, he was someone the rich and powerful knew to both rely on and fear; a self-described "problem solver," for clients he was so invested in, he regarded them as family. And he was also experienced in re-abduction cases of children...

And so, I too became family. I started a long distance correspondence with Anthony Pellicano. We talked for months about the children, what I needed to do and document to move forward. He was always available. He became a very good friend. He understood how I felt. He knew exactly what steps we should take. He counseled me, held my hand through the process; he hired people in Quito, Ecuador to search for Diane and the children. He also wanted to be sure I was ready for the re-abduction, no room for mistakes, just one bite at the apple he said. Diane was not expecting me to show up in Quito, she had not hired an attorney nor had she filed at claims in court for custody.

She was a complete fugitive on the run, deep in a South American Country, lawless in itself. She had unofficial support from Luis, and no known connections to Quito or South America for that matter beyond him. She had family in Germany and a few remaining friends in Chicago. I was hunting her and she was on the run, because she had my daughters.

Pellicano wanted a $125,000 cash retainer to go down and re-abduct the children in Quito, Ecuador. I redeemed educational bonds for college I had purchased when the girls were born, as well as stocks belonging to me. The next step was to convince the bank to release the money in a lump sum all at once. The bank officer at the bank helped me pack a suitcase with $125,000 in cash. I boarded a plane at Chicago O'Hare Airport in the morning and delivered the suitcase to him in person in Los Angeles. Nervously, I had traveled via a nonstop flight with the brief case containing the money, not something I did every day. I met and handed over the money to Detective Pellicano. He spent a few minutes talking with me, was very pleasant, and explained he would visit Quito in the near future. His contacts there were close to identifying Diane.

I became very familiar with Step 11, "Sought through prayer and meditation to improve our conscious contact with God as we understood Him, praying only for knowledge of His will for use and the power to carry that out." From my office at UIC and home, each day I took a step, made some contact or visit, to maintain my conscious contact with a power greater than myself. He answered my prayers one step at a time, one day at a time. I had little power on my own; my daughters were thousands of miles away. I had been rendered powerless, far away from another world. The key was for me to maintain a conscious contact, which I did by attending AA meetings, meeting with my sponsor, working the 12 Steps, and reading *The Big Book of Alcoholics Anonymous.*

Diane never made serious allegations against me that I was an unfit parent or unstable person, other than I was controlling and trying to keep her from the children. I was not trying to prevent her from remaining in their lives. I did want to protect the children from Diane's moods, temper, outbursts, and immaturity. So I continued the fight.

However, Pellicano notified me he had men in Quito who thought they'd spotted Diane and the children. Previously I had paid Detective Rizzo in Quito who did not find her, though it was for considerably less money. Even if I did locate her, I did not have the power or know how to re-abduct them back to the U.S. from a South American country. I couldn't imagine showing up by myself to try to persuade Diane to return to the U.S. or asking the Quito police to arrest Diane and release the children to me. Nor did I think I could overpower Diane and just walk away with children. It's not that easy to return children from South America, I correctly reasoned. Try it sometime as I did. I think you will do a lot of praying; asking for the power to carry it out.

Another detail I had to contend with: passports to move the children from country to country were needed. Diane had possession of their true passports. The question was, how would I be able to retrieve them from Ecuador or Peru without these proper credentials? I took my dilemma to a photo shop near where I lived. I had in my possession recent photos of the girls that were approximately the size of a passport photo. The shop created photos to look like actual passport photos. The girls were 7 and 8 years old at the time of their abduction. The photos were not perfect replica of passport photos, but did portray their actual appearance.

I took these photos to the U.S. Immigration Office in Chicago to obtain new passports with new copies of their birth certificates I had obtained from the State of New York. I recall the look on the Immigration Officers face as he scrutinized the images and me, and approved the new passports. Thankfully, he accepted my explanation that I had lost the previous passports. This was a gigantic step in my legal return of my daughters. Now I had a court order verifying I had permanent sole custody of my daughters, Diane was in contempt of court, with a national arrest warrant, and her passports of the children were rendered invalid with my newly acquired ones.

Soon enough, Pellicano told me to board a plane to Miami, and wait in a hotel for his signal to fly to Quito. He was timing the re-abduction of the children with my exact arrival. He had men stationed on the ground in the neighborhood where Diane lived and the children attended school. I didn't have to wait long before I received a call from him. He said to book the flight to Quito. Before I knew it, I was on the plane to South America. Landing in Quito was tricky, not something I knew about in advance of my flight. The captain warned us, "We may not be able to land because of the currents," and that he wouldn't truly know until we approached the ground. As if it was meant to be, the plane ultimately descended. I was in Quito by the evening. I took a cab to a five star hotel in the middle of what seemed to be the ghetto.

I immediately met with Detective Pellicano in his hotel room. He showed me a video and asked me to identify Diane. "Can you say this woman is her?" She was walking on the sidewalk. It was not the clearest picture, but I could definitely say it was her, especially by her distinctive gait and build. He gave me instructions to take a limousine to meet the children while they were walking home from school in the afternoon the next day.

I woke up the next morning on the phone with the U.S. Congressman Rod Blegorvich and the U.S. Ambassador for Ecuador. "He's an outstanding father and American citizen," Blegorvich advocated. "Please help him to return his daughters back home soon. He is working with Private Detective Anthony Pellicano." We hung up with the Ambassador agreeing to assist me. Things were moving at such fast pace at this time. Pellicano had everything planned. I just had to follow his orders.

As I was sitting in the limousine, my heart stopped. I caught a glimpse of my daughters walking on the sidewalk, coming home from school. One of the men directed me, "You get one of the them, I'll get the other." I jumped out of the car and ran over to Kate who burst into tears when she saw me. I immediately scooped her up and carried her to the limo. The man carried Anya to the car, and both were next to me within minutes of my spotting them. A woman on the street who witnessed the re-abduction screamed as we sped away. Kate stopped crying, while Anya was slower to respond. I asked them how they were, they didn't answer.

Not long after we arrived at my hotel room, two representatives from the U.S. Consulate in Quito met with us. They talked with the two girls and me. I showed them my court order and arrest warrant. Again, assent to the power of the law. I showed the girls pictures drawn by their classmates in the Bakewell Elementary school, and basketball cards of Michael Jordan and their other favorite professional basketball players. The girls and I had watched Jordan and the Chicago Bulls win National Basketball Association championships year after year in Chicago.

Kate said she wanted to go home right away to the

U.S. officials. With coaxing from Kate, Anya said yes as well, though she didn't want to leave her mother behind. We were all in agreement it was time to go home, finally. Both the girls knew they would not see their mother for a long time. The Consulates explained we would be escorted to a protected area at the airport and according to Pellicano's plan, I would fly to the Dominican Republic to wait for a morning flight to Miami. There were no more direct flights that day. Everyone thought it was best for us to get out of Quito before Diane could take action to stop us. So we did.

While all these preparations took place, Pellicano had arranged for the Quito police to arrest and jail Diane under the pretense she had not applied for a visa to be in Ecuador. She had been staying illegally in the country. A bit of a bribe was sufficient for the police to enforce this law. Diane remained a fugitive throughout her stay in South America. She now paid for her disregard of the law, while I continued to benefit from the power it. Pellicano said he spoke with her at the airport, and she was visibly shaken. She must have known it would be a long time before she would see the girls again. I felt sad, not triumphant, I recognized too that the girls would be separated from their mother for quite some time. Nobody was happy, but not everyone was sad.

As we took off from the plane, Anya held a picture of Diane I had taken when we lived in Nyack, NY. She grabbed it tightly and stared pensively. She too was saying goodbye. I tried to console her. She looked melancholy as she sat next to me. We landed at night in the Airport in The Dominican Republic. Dominican Republic was about midway between Quito and Miami, a dogleg to the right. We were the only ones in the airport at the midnight hour.

That night, I worried that Diane would show up and

try to reclaim the girls. That feeling would never leave me. I would always be on alert. I would frequently panic during the early years after the girls returned home. I can still see the large empty room at the airport. The girls slept on the benches. I did not want to be caught off guard, so I stayed awake. It seemed as if time stood still. I imagined that Diane and Luis would show up and demand I release the girls. I sat on the edge of the bench. Constantly scanning. Finally, when morning arrived, we started boarding the American Airlines plane, heading for Miami. Still, I was wary of everyone. We sat together as we would, for years to come. And I watched, watched, watched.

When the plane landed in Miami, I began to feel out of reach. I had left the deep recesses of South America, and far away from Diane and Luis. I had permanent, sole custody of my daughters, and we could start a new life. The girls looked gaunt, deprived, and had sallow features, reflecting their barren physical and emotional life in Quito. Diane had little money, and the girls said they had eaten mostly rice. They attended a school in Quito, and were learning Spanish. They had not told anyone they had been abducted. They were frightened. They didn't want their mother to be arrested. I learned Diane had lied to them about where they were going when they left Germany. Yet they knew something was wrong. Like little captured soldiers they followed their mother's commands. And their mother led them into the poverty stricken streets of Quito. As usual, I just took the next steps of recovery, after our return.

The girls left for Germany in July 1997. And I returned with them in February 1998. We resumed our life in the condominium in Chicago. The girls were glad to be home but for the next year, were irritable, physically and emotionally depleted. I reentered them in Bakewell Elementary School and right out of the gate, was already battling with the new principal. Diane had made friends with a teacher there, and so I was concerned she would have contact with her. I approached the principal about this, who thought I was a nut case for worrying about this teacher. I had worried about other individuals who knew Diane, and one by one I vetted them. I had to feel secure or hold back. I was constantly in fear of re-abduction for some time. As I had been warned by the police and private detectives, I would always need to remain on guard for it.

I read where anger was the prime motivator for parental abduction. The U.S. Department of Justice states in "Early Identification of Risk Factors for Parental Abduction," that,

> Compared with the general adult population, the high-conflict, litigating families and abducting families demonstrated similarly, higher levels of anger, lower levels of cooperation, a pervasive distrust of the ex-partner's parenting, greater emotional distress, and behaviors indicative of character disorders. This signaled that anger and spite, which are more often attributed to separation and divorce, were not sufficient in themselves to motivate abduction.

According to The International Parental Child Abduction Recovery Services,

> The underlying cause of child abductions in most cases is not the love for the child, but the wish for power, control, or revenge. It is therefore logical that one common personality trait of the abducting parents is that they are usually the control freaks, while the parents left behind are the calm ones. Some of the abducting parents are actually so narcissistic, that they do not understand

that their children aren't separate entities from themselves. They hold the belief that since they themselves hate the other parent, the child also hates them.

In "Parental Abduction: A Review of the Literature," the Office of Juvenile Justice and Delinquency Prevention writes that,

> One of the primary obstacles to the recovery of parentally abducted children is the general public's perception that children are not at risk of harm if they are in the physical custody of a parent, even if the parent is an abductor. Even many law enforcement personnel view parental abduction as "civil in nature" and a private family matter that is best handled outside the realm of the criminal justice system.

Attorney at Law and published author on international child abduction, Amy Savoie, J.D., Ph.D., explains,

> Several publications have described that narcissism is a personality trait that increases the risk of parental abduction. Narcissists often rationalize their violation of court orders and feel no remorse if they bend the rules to benefit themselves [...] and have difficulty controlling their anger. Eleanor Payson, a licensed family therapist, describes this nightmare as "a private one that can only be stopped by outside validation." A child raised by a narcissistic parent must grow up quickly, repressing his or her true feelings in order to serve the narcissist's needs. Moreover, the abduction of a child can have a devastating effect upon the economic well being of the left behind parent, which in turn can increase the parent's level of anxiety. Some found that the mean cost of searching for an abducted child was more than $8,000 in domestic cases and more than $27,000 in international cases. A study of

international abductions found that parents spent an average of $33,500 to search for and try to recover an abducted child. More than half of parents across all income brackets reported spending as much as or more than their annual salaries in attempting to recover their children.

I spent thousands to pay my lawyer though she failed to prevent the abduction by not objecting to Diane's vacation so soon after the divorce. By definition, Diane posed a high risk for international child abduction. She was angry, had no family relationships in the U.S., involved with a foreign citizen, she had no substantial career holding her, and did not want to or could not share the children's future, education, financial responsibilities, religion. We differed on all counts.

In addition to my attorney's fees, I paid for Private Detective Services $125,000 to Anthony Pellicano who delivered on his promises, and $10,000 to Ernie Rizzo who also delivered on his promises as well. (Though the latter chose not to continue his search in Ecuador, as he feared for his safety in the hostile South American Country.) I also had travel expenses to Germany, and many expenses that came along to facilitate my efforts.

In the end, I calculated the total costs to be in the neighborhood of $300,000 for the ultimate return of my daughters. I paid cash for these expenses from investments I made for the girls' college education, and other investments. While I am a physician, this amount certainly set me back, as I could not afford it. Do I think it was worth it? Absolutely, yes. Would I do it again? Yes, in a heartbeat. Do I think it was excessive? Probably not, except for my attorney. Expert and dedicated professionals were required for the return of my daughters. Not just anyone could do that. And they command those fees in their practice. These are market rates for these services. And I was certainly in a vulnerable position, even exploitable. Imagine those who were also in my position, but didn't have the funds?

While I had successfully negotiated a sum of money in settlement of my wrongful termination and defamation lawsuit, I had no job. The Chair needed an executor who wanted me out probably for personal and political reasons. To this day, I don't fully understand it, though I continue to believe it was arbitrary and executed on false basis. UIC paid for a 9-month salary and I agreed to not sue or be employed by them in the future. I recall in a meeting with the Chair and this faculty member, and the University's attorney, that I became very angry and lost some cool. I was not able to overcome my raw feelings about not having my employment renewed at a time when my children were lost in South America, and I needed income to support their re-abduction and myself. It didn't matter that I developed viable clinical programs, medical student and resident educational programs, as well as a fellowship in addiction psychiatry. It didn't matter I was published extensively in the medical literature, and academic books. I was a pawn in the power politics of a medical school, not my strong suit.

I was again on the short end of the proverbial stick without protection because someone didn't like me and I was viewed as a threat. My work in addictions was not popular and always posed a risk to many. People who used alcohol and drugs, particularly, addicting prescription medications had me on their radar. Users were suspicious and threatened by me because they feared I would expose them, that I'd accuse them of wrongdoing. I was a lightning rod, on whom the addicted projected their feelings of guilt and self-condemnation. Those who work in addictions were immoral, freaks, and sources of hostility from those who were judgmental regarding addictions.

Countertransference and transference pertain to all of the negative feelings surrounding addictions. In psychoanalytic theory, countertransference occurs when the therapist begins to project his own unresolved conflicts onto the client. Freud, in 1910, was the first to discuss this topic. In transference, the individual is projecting their feelings, values, judgments and thoughts on the other, whether real or imagined, true or false. Countertransference is the counter projection of feelings, values, judgments and thoughts onto the transferring party.

Since addicts are deemed immoral, those who treat the addicts are immoral. Addicts feel immoral, and the treatment provider is the target for these immoral feelings. As a doctor treating addicts, I am subjectively judged. I am immoral. I am condemned. I am estranged. I am poorly integrated. I am marginalized. I am expelled. I am an orphan in the medical profession. Countertransference and transferences would plague me for my entire career. It's like being discriminated against without legal protection. Countertransference and transference would follow me in good and bad ways in the future.

There were other faculty whose careers were in jeopardy and under similar circumstances as I, but they had tenure. Tenure gave them due process. Academic tenure is real property, and the right to possess the property. In employment contracts, particularly of public employees like school teachers or professors, it's a guaranteed right to a job (barring substantial inability to perform or some wrongful act) once a probationary period has passed. Tenure is unique to educational settings. Attaining tenured status usually means two things: first, it conveys an enhanced level of protection for academic freedom, grounded in the conviction that knowledge creation and expression of ideas should be free from intimidation or retaliation. Second, it provides an elevated form of job security.

Generally speaking, tenured professors can be dismissed only for serious misconduct or severe economic necessity. Since I had no tenure, I had no protection. The heir apparent had to act to prevent my obtaining tenure to get rid of me before it became too hard. He already had too many enemies who were tenured faculty he couldn't move. He didn't want another one. The question of tenure would continue to haunt me for years to come.

During my finals days at UIC and the re-abduction of my daughters, I had secured a position in the Department of Psychiatry at Michigan State University in East Lansing, Michigan. I also had the opportunity to work as a faculty member in Grand Rapids, Michigan, at the Pine Rest Christian Mental Health Services. I could have lived in my hometown, and the girls could have attended the same schools I had attended. I chose the home of MSU instead because I wanted to be in the mainstream of academia, and Grand Rapids was a clinical position mostly, with some supervision of medical students. Not too much academic substance. I had already established an academic career in teaching and writing to carry the message, and advance my mission to diagnosis and treat those with addictive diseases. What I didn't realize was how hard that mission would be and that so many would oppose integrating addictions into mainstream medicine and society.

The moral and judgmental attitudes for addictions permeated the public and medical profession, and formed a repellant wall around the suffering addict and alcoholic. Woefully, I learned that penetrating this wall would be fraught with risks and misunderstandings. No other field of medicine carries with it as much lack of objectivity. Common sense does not apply. And the addict controls.

My mission to carry the message to the still suffering addict will be aid and abetting by an endless stream of enablers, the medical profession as a leader. My daughters would come to know and call me as "Dr. No." On the other hand, I came to think of myself as "Dr. No" to death, and "Dr. Yes" to life, liberty, and the pursuit of happiness. I live to tell this story.

> "I respectfully submit to you that they have not found an enterprise, or that there was a common purpose [of the prosecutors' claims that Mr. Pellicano, headed a criminal enterprise.] There was an investigative agency run by a guy who'd been around a long time.
>
> I guess I could sit up here and discuss things that the government said and go over testimony, but Mr. Pellicano instructed me not to do that. And you know when Mr. Pellicano instructs you to do something, you do it."
>
> —Anthony Pellicano
>
> Representing himself at his trial, May 1st 2008
> (Pellicano v. United States District Court
> for the Central District of Los Angeles)

PART III.
WHAT IT IS LIKE NOW

15

GREATEST GIFTS,
RETURN TO ROOTS

"Success is Dependent on Effort." —Sophocles

I had a spiritual awakening as a result of the 12 Steps. I also had just completed an eight-month whirlwind tour around the world to find and retrieve my daughters, from first to third world countries, Western Europe to South America. Where I had interacted with foreign governments and diplomats, Senators, Congressman, U.S. State Department, World Renown Private Detectives, Chicago Police, German Courts, U.S. and Ecuadorian Immigrations, and many others, in my adventures to return my children.

I had had no prior experiences for my date with Lima. I had met an attractive Swiss German citizen on a train in Munich, Germany, traveling through the Alps, to Zurich, Switzerland. My daughters were born in New York, the origin of my father before moving to Chicago. After a long and contentious custody battle, Diane drew me to Peru and Ecuador, South America, and back to the scene of the agony and ecstasy, victories and defeats, in Chicago, USA. Now on to a homely place and a safe harbor of protection in the Midwest: East Lansing, Michigan.

Before moving, I took the girls to East Lansing to look for a house. We met with a realtor who himself was in the AA program and was gay. He seemed to get along well the girls, and showed us several homes, new and old. I wanted us to feel comfortable and secure in our new surroundings. Kate and Anya picked a house that needed a lot of work. They thought it was a mansion. I liked it because it was in an older neighborhood and across the street from the school they would attend. I wouldn't have to worry about transportation or long walks to school where they were vulnerable to re-abduction. Forever ready, I never took my eye off the girls, always knew where they were, what they were doing, whom they were with. The price of continuing conflict was continuing vigilance. I would live in impending fear and anxiety until the girls were 18 years old. At 18, they would be considered legally adults, and not under my legal control.

As I'd been advised, re-abduction by Diane was always a real threat to me. Call it post-traumatic stress disorder. Though she remained far way in Lima, Peru with her boyfriend Luis, I couldn't shake the idea she would boldly show up some day and try to surreptitiously capture the girls or start a legal battle by filing for custody. Again, I had the law on my side, having permanent sole custody of both Kate and Anya, and having an outstanding warrant for her arrest. Nonetheless, I had a pervasive and persistent fear of impending re-abduction by Diane or some accomplice. I remained ever vigilant, informing schools, teachers, coaches, friends, parents. It's funny; nobody ever asked many questions. Particularly, if I showed them the legal documents.

I enrolled them in the elementary school across the street, Kate in fourth grade, and Anya in third grade. It wasn't long before I got a phone call from the principal that Kate was suspended for fighting, with a boy no less. The boy in question stood out as someone looking for trouble, but Kate was not in the mood for avoiding him. For most of Kate's school career, she was an irritant to peers and teachers. She didn't like to show open respect if she didn't feel it was owed. Her saving grace was she was a good student, who greatly excelled and actually strove for higher goals in concert with her teachers. She took challenging math courses to push herself beyond her comfort levels. She became very competitive and did not fear failure.

Anya was less on edge, and did not have lofty goals. She was content with just getting by or a bit better. She did not have conflicts with friends and did not have high expectations for her friends or school. She did show early signs of talent in art and later the budding disposition of a passionate artist.

Practicing the 12 Steps had brought the return of my daughters, now I had the challenge of raising them by myself. But that fit in with my overall grandiosity that I could accomplish almost anything if I decided to do it, the bigger, the better, the more difficult, the more interesting. I can't tell you I worked from a script or had a clear map of where I would take them other than a blueprint from my upbringing. I had a few abiding principles to work from, founded on the principles from my recovery. I continued to attend AA meetings on a weekly basis, as I did not want to relapse. But I also wanted good, orderly direction, which spelled God. I had recovered from drug and alcohol addiction, and from children's abduction. I had now the opportunity to recover from job loss, perhaps my most imposing challenge.

Joy of living is the theme of the Twelfth Step. Raising my daughters was the best thing that ever happened to me, except my sobriety. I had no greater joy. I can't say it was easy, and not without good and bad times. But next to recovery, the girls took priority over whatever else I did in my life. I had moved to a community that was supportive and family oriented. I wanted the girls to live in one place for a prolonged period of time to avoid frequent moving house to house, school to school, as I did as a child. My mother lived an hour away so she too could spend time with the girls.

Action is its keyword, culminating in Step 12. Giving that asks no reward. Love that has no price tag. What is spiritual awakening? A new state of consciousness and being is received as a free gift. Readiness to receive this free gift lies in practice of the 12 Steps. The magnificent reality was I had two beautiful, precious daughters to raise, and a career to continue in a relatively recognized, challenging environment. Along with myself, I was always trying to change others, and was willing to take risks.

I had a job at the medical school at Michigan State University. I knew enough about Department of Psychiatry and MSU to know danger lurked. The Chair at the time supported Addiction Medicine, but as I later found out, he was not a permanent fixture. I met with opposition early on that did not abate. When my hiring Chair left MSU for another position, I was unprotected again, no tenure, and certainly without political support.

What about the practice of these principles in *all* our affairs? In my case, monotony, pain, and calamity from the girls' abduction turned to good use by practice of The Steps. I had had plenty of opportunity to practice these principles up to now to succeed with my international challenges. *Growing spiritually was the answer to my problems.* Placing spiritual growth first. Domination and overdependence on others would not work, and would only invite resentment and retaliation. I had to place my life on give-and-take basis with my daughters and others. More than ever I had to stay away from a drink and drug one day at a time. My daughters had only me to depend on for their safety. And I had to depend on Higher Power as necessary to recovery of from my alcoholism and drug addictions. "Practicing these principles in *all* our affairs," was the ultimate challenge I had to accept to stay sober. I had to develop a measure of humility about my feelings about personal importance. Importantly, I had to restore my instincts to their true purpose. Understanding is key to right attitudes, and right action the key to good living.

The girls had started to play soccer in Chicago, and I continued their play in East Lansing, at first in recreational leagues, then in the Club and Premier Leagues. I became the team manager for their teams as an involved parent. I had learned from my struggles with Diane that the girls profited most by two involved parents even if we were disagreeing. The key was involvement. I also loved sports and competition and enjoyed watching the girls play. As a team manager and parent, we traveled and attended games, and thus were together a good deal of the time. I became basketball coach for Kate's recreation team as well. We had a perfect 8-0 season.

It became apparent at an early age that Kate possessed athletic ability, and speed she inherited from her mother. Importantly, she also had a very competitive nature passed on from me. Anya did not have the same competitive drive, and was as slow footed as I was. Yet she participated in team sports as well, sometimes reluctantly. Her interests in team sports were more social than competitive, still an important experience. I thought team sports were especially good for girls, to train them for the competitive nature of the workplace and to establish independence. I was also acutely aware I was an older parent who would not live long into their lives, so I wanted them to be able to take care of themselves.

Kate launched into athletic prominence. She played highly competitive soccer in the Premier Leagues, and basketball in the AAU leagues. She was a star player on her high school teams in soccer and basketball, making All State in soccer. She led her high school basketball teams to League and District Championships. She showed her speed, athleticism, and competitiveness in sports. I continued to be involved on a personal level with the girls and with sports. It only deepened our connection over the years. We had many joyous hours together traveling to cities for tournaments.

Kate started to show signs of her genetic background. At the age of 16, she went to a school function in her freshman year of high school after having drunk considerable amounts of alcohol with a friend. She was apprehended by school officials and brought home. She was suspended from school and an important soccer game against a top team. I went to the principal to discuss her consequences. This demonstration came unexpectedly, and caught me surprised.

Up to this time I had not revealed to the girls my identity as an alcoholic and in recovery in AA. I cannot explain why exactly. I can tell you that the times my alcoholism became an issue were when I made it one. It was always a tough call when to reveal or not reveal my anonymity as an alcoholic. Kate's demonstrated loss of control and poor judgment over alcohol open the door. I took her to an open AA meeting where I gave a talk about my addiction and recovery. An open meeting is where a nonalcoholic can attend a meeting with alcoholics, as opposed to closed meetings where only those who have a desire not to drink, generally alcoholics, attend.

Later when Kate applied to medical school, she thanked me for discouraging her from consuming alcohol. She revealed she chose not to attend the school prom with her friends who were planning to drink. They eventually were convicted as minors in possession of alcohol, a conviction Kate did not want to explain on her medical school application. Unfortunately, there were other times I had to pick up Kate because she was intoxicated with her friends. Some may go on to develop serious problems later in life with drugs and alcohol.

While I do not have direct confirmation, I believe my younger daughter, Anya may have become involved with drugs. There were times she appeared very moody, withdrawn, and acted strangely. She also developed somewhat of a reputation in school for using marijuana that I was not aware of. She also became acquainted with a good circle of friends, so I was not overly suspicious or worried.

Here I am, a national drug expert and can't tell if my daughters are using drugs and alcohol. Her use could have explained her moods, disorganization, and inconsistent performance in school. She was however, elected to serve on the Homecoming Court, something Kate's personality prevented her from accomplishing. Both girls were attractive and outgoing. And were well known and popular in high school. Most importantly, good students, headed to good colleges, and good careers.

But peer pressure was strong. I realized earlier in my rearing of the children's lives that peers influenced their behaviors greatly. My job was to select and direct them to the proper peers to help them to stay out of harm's way, and to make the most for them. In a sense, the peers raise your children. As Friedrich Nietzsche said, "The surest way to corrupt a youth is to instruct him to hold in higher esteem those who think alike than those who think differently."

Peer pressure is commonly associated with risk behaviors, and is a strong predictor of an adolescent's own behavior. Peer pressure can be positive or negative. In my case, my daughters were influenced and supported by strong peers, but did not always follow their lead. I steered them in the direction of peers with behaviors that I thought were desirable and most productive for the short and long haul. Kate's selection of peers had parents who would communicate with me, and I drove Kate crazy because I talked with other parents. She said, "You have no right to talk with other parents," but that certainly limited undesirable behaviors and outcomes for her and peers. Anya didn't like it much either but my communications with other parents had similar effects on her behaviors as well. Wikipedia explains that,

> Peer pressure is widely recognized as a major contributor to the initiation of substance use, particularly in adolescence This has been shown for a variety of substances, including nicotine and alcohol. While this link is well established, mediating factors do exist. Parental monitoring is negatively associated with substance use; yet when there is little monitoring, adolescents are more likely to succumb to peer coercion during initiation to substance use, but not during the transition from experimental to regular use. Peer pressure was a factor leading to heightened risk in the context of social gatherings, little parental monitoring, and if the individual reported themselves as vulnerable to peer pressure. Conversely, some research has observed that peer pressure can be a protective factor against substance use.

My monitoring of their alcohol and drug use had some positive effects on Kate and Anya. But it didn't matter that I was a national expert on drugs and alcohol to them. As adolescents I didn't know anything period, let alone about drugs and alcohol, after all their friends did it so it must be ok, no matter what I said.

Substance use is likely not attributed to peer pressure alone. Evidence of genetic predispositions for substance use exists. With my family history, I certainly provided them with heavy genetic loading. Just as my appearance was evident in how they looked, so did I biologically influence their attraction to and risk for alcohol and drug use. Peer pressure produces a wide array of negative outcomes. Substance use was also predicted by peer pressure susceptibility such that greater susceptibility was predictive of greater alcohol and drug use.

As the sole male parent and provider, mothers became my best friends and social life. I extended my theory that an involved parent helped the girls in school life, and I had regular communications with the teachers. Grades were paramount, and as my parents did to me, I drilled into the girls that good performance in school was the key to their success in life.

Kate was naturally interested in school and obtained good grades. She was very organized and had a knack for knowing just how much she had to work to excel. She did not like to overdo studying. Anya was not particularly organized, though interested in school, she did not value grades or academic achievement as much. She had to be reminded to turn in work. She lacked considerable confidence. I, of course, was not a particularly good role model for high school, but I expected more from them. I didn't want them to expect to manipulate their way through academics as I did.

As the girls moved into their teen-age years, I experienced mounting challenges and stress. When they were younger I felt I was always a step behind in figuring out what was happening, good or bad, and scrambled to develop a strategy to deal with it. Their adolescence was perhaps the greatest challenge I had next to my battle with drugs and alcohol.

Adolescence is a rapid transitional state. Vicissitudes of adolescence are successive, alternating, changing phases or conditions, as of life or fortune; ups and downs: regular change or succession of one state or thing to another, change; mutation; mutability. The struggle for independence from versus dependence on parents is obvious during adolescence. The teenagers' manner in this struggle is crude and offensive sometimes. I can remember many episodes of defiance in the girls, and ample profanities to project their efforts to establish autonomy from me.

The paradox is that the girls often commented that I did not micro manage their lives, and did not ask them to report their private activities or inner thoughts. Nonetheless they felt the need to express their belligerence towards me on a pretty regular basis. I can recall frequent shouting matches over pretty simple things, and their refusal to submit to my requests or orders. Their objections often made little sense, but they viewed me as controlling and interfering. They wanted their independence but did not want me to protect them from the responsibilities or consequences of their decisions, good or bad. Their school performance was their business but my having regular contact with teachers definitely had a positive influence on their progress. Without it, the grades would suffer, and their attention and focus would wander. Curiously, they did respond to my "butting in" with improvement.

I did not have romantic relationships with women while I raised the girls. I am uncertain why, but I know I did not want to reintroduce more problems for them from outside relationships with women. I was also still shell shocked from my previous relationship with Diane, and did not relish more battles over the girls. I don't believe I had more than a date or two during our years together.

I continued to attend AA, though I started to struggle with going to meetings. I did not want to hear others, forced myself to listen, developed resentments against them. But I maintained that desire not to drink, and continued to attend meetings. I relied on my discipline from years of working the program. In my 39 years of sobriety and abstinence from alcohol and drugs, I don't think I missed attending a meeting in a week or 7 days. A string I try to keep come hell or high water, and able to do so blessed with good health. Times I had surgery, I asked AA members to hold a meeting in my house, or I made it to a meeting in less than perfect shape.

Believe it or not we did not discuss their mother or the child abduction much over the years. I lamented at times that despite our disagreements, her anger, and my controlling manner, Diane's involvement in the girls' lives would have been preferable to my raising them alone. That's not to say they did not respond to me, just that I felt the loss of their mother was hard to accept despite her selfish and unilateral disruptive actions. I cannot fully assess to this day what long lasting impact their abduction and consequent loss of mother had on them. After their recovery, I could not see a long lasting change in their personalities and moods. They had strengths and vulnerabilities from childhood that persisted into adulthood. I could not discern drastic departures from predictable and expected courses over their lives.

I had taken the girls to University of Michigan football games from a very young age. As we walked across the famous "Diag" on campus during a football Saturday, I said to them, "This is where you will go to college." And Kate blurted out, "No." Which I took that to mean, "Not without my mother's consent."

We continued to attend games over the years even when we lived in Chicago. Kate had many opportunities for college because of her outstanding academic record and prowess as a soccer and basketball player. She was accepted at the University of Chicago, New York University, and other notable schools. However, her approach was typical of her belligerence. We attended an orientation day at the University of Michigan, and she was profane about her experience. Meanwhile, I was taken in by the experience, and felt a profound connection to the University.

Kate was interviewed by the U-M soccer coach and considered for a preferred walk on for the team. Which wasn't too bad considering that full scholarships were hard to come by in that sport. Eventually Kate was accepted to Michigan and did attend. After she graduated, she said she would have her children attend Michigan—she liked it so much.

Before the semester began, I remember when we bought her books for her freshman year of college. Though she did not declare it to me, she enrolled in premedical courses. Surprisingly, or not, she did pretty well her freshman year and decided to advance in her premedical studies. She also joined and was active in a sorority on campus. And fun for me, she played U-M Club Soccer for three years. I attended many of her games, including National tournaments in Florida, and Arizona. She was a star forward who had a knack for scoring goals. Kate then decided to apply for medical school, and was accepted to Wayne State University. After graduation, she entered a residency in General Surgery. Her determination never wavered. Once again, she followed her dad's footsteps in medicine, but did better than I did. I had to use pull and influence to get into medical school, whereas she gained her way in on her own merit and achievement. No outside influence. She was sober, I was drunk. She showed up for her work, I did not. She had remained in the one location, whereas I had moved frequently. She was hopeful, I was hopeless. We did share in common, an unwavering persistence.

Anya often followed her sister, so she applied and was accepted as a student at the University of Michigan a year later. She entered their school of Art and Design and spent several summers at Interlochen and Blue Lake Art Camp. Anya had found her calling as a talented artist in high school. She was also well rounded like her sister and played sports in high school. But she had a rough time with her moods and teachers.

She was irritable, very anxious, and spent long hours refining her art projects. She was resistant to her teachers' interventions. She struggled with the Art School's abstract orientation and philosophy. She wanted more practical, hands on instructions. While her focus became metals and jewelry, she excelled at painting. Her grades were stellar in drawings and paintings, whereas her performance in the more conceptual tasks were criticized. Her senior project was remarkable, but was graded down because she did not engage in the all-important process.

I like to think her creative nature fought for expression and authenticity. Her artistic integrity was more important than burdensome steps in a process. She was really an individualist who wanted to express her ideals and unique objects for others to enjoy. She followed my individualism and defiance, unwillingness to compromise. She persisted whereas I wavered, due to my drunkenness, or she may have succumbed to intoxication like me. She was driven by creativity. I was driven by destructive drugs.

It was at this time when I was losing my individual spiritual awakening, and did not carry the message well when working with other alcoholics. I struggled at meetings, did not want to go, did not want to listen to others' testimonials. I persevered on grit and discipline along with determination. I never lost sight of the desire to drink. But I watched the clock until the meeting ended. I continued to pray, perfunctorily, dutifully, without passion. My level of internal stress and exhaustion wore on my enthusiasm and spiritual energy. But I remembered how it was, and I did not want to go back to the hell of drinking and drugging.

I now had the singular purpose of raising my daughters, and I was focused on that responsibility. Perhaps in my heart they became a higher importance than my recovery. But I learned early on that I had to have my priorities in order; staying sober in AA was first and necessary, as all other priorities were contingent on my sobriety.

My family and personal life came second, and I naturally gravitated to that priority more as I became the sole custodial parent. I was there for Kate and Anya 24 hours a day, seven days a week. I negotiated with them, no one else. I could not pass them off to anyone else. I could not let work or something else interfere with my responsibilities to the girls. I had their lives in my grasp, and I planned their lives with them. I did not know the outcomes for them exactly, but I knew the steps for them to take one day at a time, and the requirements to get them where they wanted to go. I knew Kate would be successful in whatever she did. I was not as confident in Anya as she did not show the same determination, but she usually came around. Friends and relatives told me I was doing a good job, was a good father. In fact, parents would look to me as an example. I was a natural, but not perfect.

What about Diane, the girls' mother? When she abducted the children, I didn't know she realized she risked losing all rights to custody and visitation. I didn't know what her attorney told her. I always felt they knew about Diane's plan to abduct the girls, though I could not prove it. Especially since she abducted them to country far from their home, South America. She may have thought it was beyond my reach. Ordinarily, I would agree. Now, I had to be ever vigilant of re-abduction.

I was advised by the police to sever any contact between the girls and Diane. I had cut ties with my own attorney. We had a conversation in which she asked for more money for her services. I decided that I had already spent a quarter of million dollars to return my daughters because she had not objected to the court Diane's taking the girls to Germany for a vacation. Had I been more sophisticated, I would have filed for legal malpractice against my attorney to retrieve my financial losses. In retrospect, I would have done that; another costly lesson. However at that time, I was not careful about money, didn't avoid debt, and had racked up large amounts of it.

Otherwise, Diane did not have contact with her daughters other than one supervised telephone conversation, arranged by my attorney, until the girls turned the age of 18. At 18, Kate and Anya were no longer legally considered children. Diane eventually moved to the U.S. when Luis was assigned to the Peruvian Consulate in Miami,

Florida. She had married him, so she benefited from diplomatic immunity, and therefore the arrest warrant was not enforceable. The girls eventually chose to make contact with her after they were of age.

Over the years, I had thought, despite the conflicts and disagreements between Diane and me regarding how to raise them, it would have been better if Diane had been a part of their lives. Don't ask me why I thought that. The girls didn't ask much about their mother, didn't want to speak with or see her, never talked about her. I rarely mentioned her positively or negatively. We had our lives together. It was definitely easier for them to not think about her. I had become their mother and father, one in the same.

At Michigan State University, I started start to work clinically on an addiction unit at St. Lawrence, developing detoxification programs and teaching programs for medical students and residents. They rotated on the unit to learn clinically how to take care of patients with addictions. The educational programs became popular, and I was bringing money into the department and providing valuable educational programs.

However, politics and prejudice prevailed over purpose and value. The promotion committee tried to terminate me for academic reasons. No rationale was given, no basis for their conclusions. I was saved at the bell by the chair Kevin Navarro who had just returned from serving as the interim Dean of the College of Human Medicine. He promptly reversed their unsubstantiated recommendations, and submitted a reinstatement for me. But not long after, he moved on to become Dean of a Medical School in Texas, and left me to the mercy of the incoming chair of the Department of Psychiatry.

My contract was not renewed by Jake Fisher, the

new Chair, who had been in the Department for years, and friends with the faculty who previously tried to axe me. I was given a year's notice and was told the Department wanted to go in a different direction. What did I take that to mean? They no longer wanted to teach addictions to the medical students and residents? I sought legal advice. Because of my experience at UIC, I had negotiated a contract I thought had contained due process before accepting the position at MSU. I had been told that I had a contract protected by a similar due process, contained in tenure. Which meant before nonrenewal of my contract, I would have a review at various levels, leading up to the Dean of the Medical School. I felt the stigma from my work in addictions contributed to my demise. At least, addiction was a low priority in the Department as it was in medicine as a whole. I could not count on my colleagues as others could. However, Jake Fisher was doing a general house cleaning in the Department, and I was on his list.

Though I had developed profitable clinical and highly rated teaching programs in addictions, led the department in the number of peer reviewed publications, was a nationally known expert, I was dispensable. I had little support and did not know how to develop it politically within the Department. MSU did not renew my contract, and gave no reason. To me, they did not follow their publicized due process, instead they disregarded and disrespected clinical and academic excellence in addictions.

Instead of simply leaving as I had in other situations, I decided to file a grievance within the college and later the university. I had lost the appeal at the college level but eventually won on appeal at the University level. My grievance was heard by my peers, and I was represented by them. Only to have the president of the University deny the committee's recommendation to reinstate me in my previous faculty positions.

As my own attorney, I then filed a lawsuit for wrongful termination in the Western Michigan U.S. District Court, alleging I had not received due process and was discriminated against based on my work in addictions. Unfortunately, I lost at the early level of summary judgment. Apparently, the Judge decided that the university could offer window dressings of due process but then make me sign a memorandum that only applied to a fixed term appointment. I in fact did not have a rolling, renewable contract subject to due process as advertised, rather all I possessed was an at will, fixed term contract, for a period of time. Stealth and politics, deceit and power, and no protection. Total disrespect for my expertise and contributions to addictions in the University. Another defeat at the institutional level. This is why I went to law school, to defend myself and sue for change.

I'm still standing
(Yeah yeah yeah)

—"I'm Still Standing" Elton John

16

OVERCOMING WITH CHANGE

*"He that will not apply new remedies must
expect new evils."* —Francis Bacon

Personally, I had now experienced the power of the law, positively. With a court order from a probate court in Chicago, I had influenced the world in the fight to get my daughters back. I learned the law is a wonderful thing if it is on your side, and can bring about change for benefit. Without that court order, I would have been just another forlorn parent in search of their lost children. I may have received sympathy and a bit of advice, but no real action or power.

Lack of power, that was my dilemma. I looked no further around me than to women and minorities, who used the law to bring about widespread change to advance their causes. They used discrimination as basis for their claims for fair and equal treatment. Because of their civil rights work, women and discriminated minorities gained legal status as "protected classes" with special consideration and affirmative action applied.

In the United States Federal Anti-Discrimination Law, a protected class is a characteristic of a person which cannot be targeted for discrimination. The following characteristics are considered "Protected Classes" by Federal Law:

- Race – *Civil Rights Act of 1964*
- Color – *Civil Rights Act of 1964*
- Religion – *Civil Rights Act of 1964*
- National origin – *Civil Rights Act of 1964*
- Age (40 and over) – *Age Discrimination in Employment Act of 1967*
- Sex – *Equal Pay Act of 1963* and *Civil Rights Act of 1964.* (The Equal Employment Opportunity Commission includes discrimination based on gender presentation and sexual orientation as protected beneath the class of 'sex'.)
- Pregnancy – *Pregnancy Discrimination Act*
- Citizenship – *Immigration Reform and Control Act*
- Familial status – *Civil Rights Act of 1968.* Title VIII: Housing cannot discriminate for having children, with an exception for senior housing
- Disability status – *Rehabilitation Act of 1973* and *Americans with Disabilities Act of 1990*
- Veteran status – *Vietnam Era Veterans' Readjust -ment Assistance Act of 1974* and *Uniformed Ser -vices Employment and Reemployment Rights Act*
- Genetic information – *Genetic Information Non-discrimination Act*

Unfair and lethal discrimination against classes of addicted individuals is evident in government policy. Inexplicably, the tobacco settlement does not stipulate that the states must use funds to treat and reduce health related consequences from smoking, despite litigation based on damages to cigarette smokers. Similarly, states can determine how much to tax, and how to spend the tax revenue from cigarette sales, without having legally to apply tax revenue to tobacco related issues. Taxation without representation, a blatant practice to ride the backs of the addicted smoker, with public and legal support to exploit addiction.

Consequently, because of the terms of the tobacco settlement and tax revenue being dependent on sales of tobacco products, there is incentive for states to implicitly encourage cigarette consumption to people at any age, particularly, impressionable young people. For the state to do otherwise would mean the tax revenues would decline correspondingly.

Across states, an average of only 6% of the tobacco settlement funding is dedicated to health related consequences from tobacco consumption, prevention, and treatment of nicotine addiction. Moreover, the State of Michigan dedicates less than 20% of tobacco tax revenue to cigarette health related consequences and prevention, and applies tobacco tax revenue mostly to non-health expenditures, such as education and general government operating expenses.

Given that 440,000 persons die annually from tobacco related use, only discriminatory practices by states could explain using settlement and tax money to fund government activities totally unrelated to the health and welfare of those already addicted to cigarettes or are at risk to become addicted. However, there is no other condition, medical or otherwise, where public policy, public health, and safety condone such a magnitude of self-destruction in the US, except discriminated minorities.

Thus, a question remains whether class action litigation for tobacco settlement was to remedy health care practices, or just perpetuate the discrimination against afflicted, powerless, addicted individuals by exploiting a funding source to support state governments. The answers are mixed from the history of class action litigation for addictions heretofore as courts have been reluctant to fully endorse class action as a superior method to traditional litigation, and find common questions predominant among individuals with drug and alcohol addictions.

Addiction is a legal and medical disease where personal choice is overcome by changes in brain chemistry that compel victims to use alcohol and addicting medications destructively. It is defined by a preoccupation with acquiring alcohol and drugs, and compulsive use and pattern of relapse despite adverse consequences. Preoccupation is demonstrated by a high priority of use, as illustrated by continuing to purchase cigarettes despite escalating taxes; compulsive use is evident in continued use, despite an annual mortality rate of over 400,000 and relapse manifested by unsuccessful attempts to remain abstinence from cigarettes despite these fatal consequences. Pervasive to these behaviors is a loss of control over drug use, seen in excessive use over time despite accumulation of morbidity and mortality. The loss of control is largely unconscious and persistent, and is similar to drive states such as hunger and sex. As with drive states, conscious control is possible, but the untreated drive state to smoke is expressed ultimately in compulsive and repetitive drug use.

Court decisions generally hold that addiction to alcohol and drugs is not willful misconduct. In addition, that being a drug addict or alcoholic is a status, and not a crime. In Robinson vs. California, the Supreme Court ruled that the California law against being a drug addict, making it a crime, was unconstitutional. As such, the Court held a law could not make "status" a crime, and the treatment for addiction represented a different goal than punishment for a crime. Moreover, in Powell vs. State of Texas, the Supreme Court held that while public drunkenness was a crime, being an alcoholic was not; rather instead, it was a status.

It really helped that I had a disease, and not a moral or character problem. I did not have to feel I was a bad person or deserved to feel shameful, for a condition I did not cause. Scientific evidence demonstrates that there are centers in the brain responsible for the addictive use of alcohol and other drugs. These addiction brain centers are similar to those responsible for other drive states in the phylogenetically older portions of the brain responsible for instincts and basic drive states such as hunger and sex. Addicting drugs including nicotine and alcohol, act on specific neuronal circuitry to stimulate reinforced use and ultimately compulsive, pathological use. Once loss of control develops, which is the cardinal manifestation of addictive disease, it remains indefinitely.

While I am not to blame for my addictive disease, I am responsible for having it. The addicted individual is responsible for the consequences of their actions while under the influence of addicting drugs through out of control use. However, they do not use addicting drugs intentionally in a pathological pattern, and often commit acts against their will, or at least unintentionally. Courts often mitigate charges and sentencing for alcoholics and drug addicts, recognizing their lack of *mens rea* or guilty mind for their actions due the influence of addictive disease.

As an alcoholic and addict myself, I understand stigma from the victim point of view. Stigma has many faces and is founded in a moral or biased judgment. In my case, I think of myself as less than, inferior, immoral under the pressure of stigma. Stigma affects both the beholder and the victim. It is irrational and negative, destructive and damaging, and counter therapeutic. How would you like to feel judged, outside, different, and condemned? You know how it is to judge someone who looks like they do it to themselves, with a disregard for others or to blame them for their troubles? We don't feel that way if someone has a disease, even if they contribute to their demise. If someone is overweight and has a heart attack, you say they had a heart attack. If someone has an addiction to alcohol, you said they did it to themselves. What is the difference? The addict is at fault, and the obese heart attack victim is not. The addict is a bad person, the heart attack victim had something bad happen to them.

I decided I could not make enough impact in helping those with drug and alcohol problems through education and publications. I had published many articles but had been a victim of discrimination in the workplace in several places. Importantly, I had not seen alcohol and drug curriculum in medical schools commensurate with their occurrence in patient populations. Out of control prescribing by physicians was increasing and causing alarming rates of addiction to drugs and alcohol. Patients were dying, and physicians prescribed narcotics freely and on demand. Also, medical schools remained delinquent and seriously deficient in education in addictions. Medicine as a whole was negligent and belligerent to practicing responsible and evidence based medicine in regards to addictions.

Addiction rates to narcotics soared. Physicians were not held accountable for dangerous prescribing, pharmaceutical profits escalated, hospitals prescribed narcotics for patient satisfaction, disability and deaths reached new heights. No one was being held accountable, except the suffering addict; who foots the bill for everyone else.

My grandiosity kicked in and I enrolled in law school to change medical practice, first part time, then graduating, preparing and taking the bar examination. At first, I just wanted to take a single course. I saw signs displaying the law school on my way to the medical school office. After visiting with an admissions officer, I was encouraged to apply to law school, not just take a course. One thing led to another, and I was accepted into the program at the age of 57.

In my mind, I had not committed to actually enrolling, as I would take it one step at a time. I was offered loans despite being an employed doctor, to add to another addictive problem I had developed, getting in debt. Concurrently, I continued to raise my daughters, work as a Professor in the medical school, act as team manager for soccer, coach for basketball, father, mother, etc.

I liked law school, and found the professor supportive and interesting. I finished in the top 25% with a little politics of buttering up with the professors. Remarkably, I had not had much experience with essay examinations but managed to learn how to answer questions with lengthy and detailed written answers. I decided my purpose in law school was to sue doctors, hospitals, and the medical profession. I had set my sights sky high. I was on a mission from God, and He would supply me with knowledge and will to succeed.

I needed to fund my law practice since plaintiff medical malpractice was contingency work. So I started working at Pine Rest as a psychiatrist on weekends, by driving 60 miles back and forth to Grand Rapids. Then, I worked in Spectrum Hospital and St. Mary's Hospital on Consultation Service. After practicing law in the morning, I drove the 60 miles in the afternoons and worked until evening, then drove back to East Lansing. I saw tons of medical and psychiatric patients prescribed addicting medications, and excessive amounts of other medications.

I started a law practice on my own, first renting a single office, then expanding my practice. I started with a law review caliber clerk who created my first case with a mistake on service which we corrected. The medical malpractice laws in Michigan were among the most difficult and prejudicial to the plaintiff. Tort reform had hit Michigan, and the law required a notice of intent to sue to be sent before the suit was actually filed.

The defense had six months to design its case before the lawsuit actually began. The idea was to encourage settlement but that was not supported in the law. The law prescribed a cap or limit on how much noneconomic damages could be awarded, so an insurance company knew its exposure to liability. Noneconomic damages were pain and suffering, and not liberally measured. Noneconomic damages were not awarded for pain and suffering from addiction, or the depression, anxiety, guilt, hopelessness, helplessness, lost relationships, moral degradation, debilitation, bewilderment.

Because of the notice of intent requirement and liability cap, insurance companies were not encouraged to settle, and found no reason to compensate injured patients. As a result, they fought every motion and case knowing that their costs would be low. Defendants could send a message to medically harmed patients that they would not be compensated unless economic damages were at stake. Economic damages were usually awarded to employed plaintiffs. Otherwise, future income was not calculated. Most patients who were victims of narcotic addictions from physician prescribing were debilitated and unemployed from the medications. Doctors who maintain patients on narcotic medications don't do justice and eventually cause harm, even permanent harm. Satisfying patients who seek and demand addicting drugs because of their addiction is not in their interests.

The first case I filed a lawsuit for involved a doctor who prescribed morphine for years to someone clearly addicted to narcotics. Constance Smith was prescribed morphine for a medical condition, paralysis from polio, which is not usually associated with pain. The polio paralysis was from childhood, and she did not need a brace but wore one on occasion to convince doctors to prescribe her morphine. She also had a history of alcoholism, which is a significant reason not to prescribe morphine.

The prescribing of morphine led her to disrupted relationships, disability, poor motivation for self-care, and neglect of her daughters. The daughters felt abandoned and punished by their mother. They tried many times to speak with her doctor to discontinue prescribing narcotics to no avail. The doctor continued to prescribe narcotics to an obviously addicted patient, despite many warnings from loved ones. The doctor had already been censored and fined by the State Medical Board for other illegal activities. He also had a mental illness that interfered with his judgment in caring for patients. Yet the State Medical Board continued to allow him to prescribe dangerous narcotic medications.

She also had breathing difficulties and was at risk for lethal overdose. Sure enough, she died of respiratory failure while taking the morphine. Her death was one of the worst kind, suffocation from depressing respiration from the narcotic suppression of breathing, this means she was gasping for her breath, frighteningly knowing the end was in sight, helpless to do anything to save herself. Of course, during the doctor's deposition, he denied everything, made up facts, acted as if she did it to herself. The deposition lasted seven hours, and his attorney tried to intimidate me, acting in a threatening manner, perhaps in response to my indignation over the doctor's absurd testimony.

The doctor actually did not think prescribing morphine did not cause addiction or breathing problems. He did everything "right." No harm to his patient. He also missed her pneumonia when he saw her just before she died. Although he documented in his notes he examined her, he never did. I doubt he even checked boxes that had made up his examinations. He had prescribed morphine for years over the objections of her family. The doctor ignored pleas by the daughters to stop his prescribing. There's no telling what he himself may have been taking. I could not get his psychiatric records.

She actually died under another doctor's care in the emergency room hours before she suffocated. She called the paramedics early in the morning when she could not breathe and was taken to the hospital. She was examined, but not admitted as she had been multiple times in the past for pneumonia and respiratory distress. She was given morphine, believe it or not, and a medication called Albuterol to help her breathing. The only problem was Albuterol masked the symptoms, and the underlying pneumonia and narcotic respiratory depression. Because of this imminent risk from morphine combined with pneumonia, she had been admitted on at least two prior occasions to the ICU for these problems to the same hospital. The Emergency Physician had access to these records. Nonetheless, she was not admitted and instead sent home. Not long after she got home, she took her morphine as prescribed by her doctors, stopped breathing, and died. The family was devastated. Their mother was gone forever.

What is sad about this case, and others like it, is that morphine is not a pain killer. In fact, morphine causes pain, paradoxically. Opioid induced hyperalgesia: algesia is perception of pain, hyper is increased pain, and analgesic is relief from pain. Morphine is supposed to be an analgesic or reduce pain. What happens is morphine eventually increases pain, even when taken as prescribed, which is a reason doctors prescribe greater amounts over time. Also, morphine is highly addicting which causes compulsive use over time, and continued use from the addiction, not pain relief, in spite of increasing pain from the morphine. Addiction is the only plausible explanation why patients continue to take a dangerous drug that is not working, and may kill them.

Many doctors don't understand addiction or hyperalgesia for that matter. Patients on chronic morphine develop disability, and other negative effects of morphine, that can only be avoided by stopping the morphine. Not to mention just how dangerous are prescribing conditions for increasing pain and highly addicting and lethal medications. Doctors are supposed to be smart, but many are not when it comes to addicting medications. Nor do they want to learn much to help their patients.

In a *Journal of Addiction Research and Therapy* article titled "Prescription Opioid Medications: Efficacy in Chronic Pain," it states that:

Addiction to prescription opioid medications is an enormous and widespread public health problem. Overdose deaths relating to opioid pain medications have increased and now exceed deaths involving heroin and cocaine combined. In 2013, there were 43,982 total drug overdose deaths in the United States. 16,235 were attributed to prescription analgesics and 6,235 were attributed to heroin. Thus, opioids accounted for 28,470 or 64.7% of all drug related deaths in 2013.

Notably, the increased rate of opioid medications prescribed has been followed by alarming increases in the negative consequences related to their pharmacological and addictive properties. These negative consequences include but are not limited to: mortality, overdose morbidity, serious adverse events, dependence/addiction, lifelong disability, and loss of family and community. For example, in 2013, 207 million prescriptions were written for prescription opioid pain medications. Prescription opioid use is also taxing on the economy. It has been estimated that medical and nonmedical use of opioid pain medications unnecessarily costs insurance companies as much as $72.5 billion a year for adverse consequences related to opioid medications.

On the 2012 list of top ten medications prescribed, three of them were Hydrocodone opioids (HYCD/APAP). There was a total of 129,068,000 prescriptions of Hydrocodone made by three different manufacturers: Actavis, Mallinckrodt, and Qualitest Products. Oxycodone prescriptions, the second most frequently prescribed opioid behind Hydrocodone, rose from 18.8% in 2007 to 24.4% in 2011 of all prescription pills dispensed.

Opioid addiction should be viewed as a chronic medical disorder, such as hypertension, schizophrenia, and diabetes. As with the other diseases, a cure is unlikely, but long-term treatment can decrease the disease's adverse effects and improve day-to-day functioning.

I naturally thought to improve physician prescribing of addicting drugs, suing them was needed. Education didn't work, doctors were not smart enough to learn about addiction. Politics to promote prescribing narcotics for pain was too strong, and obliterated the public health issues of lack of efficacy and dangerousness of narcotic drugs like morphine. And today's public loves addiction, particularly, to drugs, sex, and rock and roll. Why did I think a court would look at narcotic medications in the medical profession any differently? I didn't care. I was going to be different. I knew so much. I still believed in justice and doing the right things. I reasoned incorrectly, that the court would want to help people, save lives, reduce suffering, right? Maybe? I found out the answers to these questions the hard way, as I often did, and still do.

As the attorney, I filed a lawsuit in a Wayne County Court. I started off in complaint, alleging that the doctor and hospital prescribing morphine and failure to admit plaintiff caused her death. That seemed logical to me, actually a self-evident truth. Anybody who knew anything about morphine and narcotics would know how dangerous they are, and that someone who can't breathe on morphine should be admitted to the hospital. Of course, I knew there were going to be a defense, but I thought they would be reasonable and see it my way. Naive? Maybe. In my first case, I had sued two defendants, the doctor who prescribed morphine, and the hospital emergency department that failed to admit plaintiff in respiratory distress. I alleged medical malpractice.

Medical malpractice starts with a doctor patient relationship that constitutes a duty owed, and that was not too hard to establish in the case of either doctor. The doctor treated the plaintiff for 10 years, and prescribed morphine the entire time up to the time of her death. The emergency physician treated and discharged the patient just prior to her death. Not only the doctor, but the hospital is vicariously liable as the acting site where the medical malpractice took place, and the physician as their representative.

The hospital has the obligation to provide reasonable care in its employees, in this case, a contract employee through an emergency physician group. Powerful, wealthy insurance companies represent and hire defense attorneys to defend the doctor against medical malpractice suits. The hospital represented and defended itself. Both insurance companies and hospitals have vast resources to intimidate and outspend plaintiff attorneys, and political backing from the public and court systems. Another problem I had was being an outsider and not in the Detroit club of attorneys. Protecting turf was a strong motivation to keep me from being successful.

The next element of a malpractice, is that the duty was breached when the provider failed to conform to the relevant standard of care, a legal term, established by an expert witness. The standard of care means the degree of care and skill of the average health care provider who practices the provider's specialty, taking into account the medical knowledge that is available to the physician. Another way to describe the term is that the standard of care is based on the customary practices of the average physician; what the average physician would customarily or typically do in similar circumstances. The standard of care is not the ideal, but based on what the reasonable, prudent physician would do under similar circumstances.

In the case of prescribing opioid medications for chronic pain, unfortunately, many physicians prescribe narcotic medications for chronic pain despite their inherent dangerousness. What is really crazy is that if the patient develops problems from the physician prescribing opioids, it is somehow deemed the patient's fault. As if the patient, not the doctor, should know better than to take a doctor prescribed medication that will harm them. Somehow the doctor is let off the hook, never held responsible for getting the patient addicted to a highly addicting medication, and the patient is blamed for becoming addicted. The doctor is supposed to have superior knowledge and exercise care in the patient's interest; never their fault.

Thus, addiction is a disease caused by the patient, willfully, intentionally, and deceitfully. While the doctor should know that an opioid is highly addicting and danger-ous as a controlled substance, the patient is the one respon-sible and to blame for any addiction and consequent harm from the medications. When the patient becomes addicted because of the physician prescribing, the physician can call on stigma and prejudice to bail them out of problems caused by the medications. If addiction is considered a moral problem, and not a disease, then the patient is guilty. Thus, it is easy to see why a judge or jury would find it easy to excuse the doctor, and find the patient at fault.

Despite the prevailing judgmental and negative attitudes, against all odds, we filed a lawsuit and alleged that the doctors and hospitals breached or failed to meet the standard of care. We alleged that they should have ex-ercised reasonable care in prescribing a dangerous medica-tion. Actually, we thought the physician owed a higher duty given the dangerousness and high mortality from narcotic medications.

What I didn't plan on, but should have, is a very biased and prejudicial judge. She hated my client, "I can't stand the name Constance Smith," and had a vendetta against my famous expert, Kurt Schneider MD. She showed highly prejudicial attitude towards me, limited the length of my opening statement, yet allowed the defense unlimited time. She blatantly approached me with disdain. She showed exaggerated reactions to me and my case, even un-provoked anger towards me and my client. As expected in an addiction case, I did not get just judicial decisions; we did not get a fair trial.

To me, it was not hard to show the breach or de-viation from the standard of care, and that the physician prescribing was a direct cause or proximate cause of the plaintiff's death. To me, all of this was a "no brainer." Had the physician not continuously, irresponsibly prescribed her morphine without valid medical indication, she would not have died. Furthermore, had the hospital not discharged the plaintiff, rather admitted her to hospital instead, she would not have suffocated from morphine asphyxiation.

The kicker in a plaintiff medical practice case is to show the doctor and hospital's actions were the proximate cause of her injury or death. Proximate cause is that their actions foreseeably caused her death. Meaning, their ac-tions were sufficiently careless, or were performed without consideration demanded by the standard of care. Again, to me it was all a "no brainer," that prescribing dangerous medications without cause, and discharging a patient in respiratory distress on morphine were careless actions that foreseeably caused her death.

In the end, I had to show that a drug addict was entitled to and deserved the same standard of care that was generally accepted for other diseases in the medical profes-sion. That was just too much for me to overcome. I could not defeat the prevailing prejudice that drug addicts were worthy of same justice and fairness afforded to other vic-tims of medical malpractice. I could not convince the judge that she should give a drug addict a break, and hold the physician and hospital responsible and liable for her death based on what they did.

The judge had demonstrated contempt for our case, and did not want her courtroom to show justice to an immoral drug addict. She ended the case early in a directed verdict, not allowing it to go to the jury. She did not even give my client and her deceased mother a full day in court. She obviously was worried that the jury might look beyond prejudice and bias, and hold the physicians responsible for their actions and malpractice.

The judge held that we did not establish proximate cause, meaning the doctor's prescribing did not cause her death, and the hospital's failure to admit did not cause her death, despite that morphine intoxication was listed as a cause of death in the medical examiner's report. To be honest, I wonder if the judge may have been using and addicted to narcotic drugs herself, as she complained about back pain and had such a personal response to our plaintiff's use of narcotic drugs

The injustice did not stop there, however. I then appealed the case to the Michigan Court of Appeals. A panel of three judges reviewed the case, and two held we did not establish a proximate cause, and left the conclusion that the plaintiff somehow killed herself. I could also read the scorn on the faces of two of the judges, who would not look me in the eye during the oral arguments. My expert had put together an intrinsic medical rationale for how morphine foreseeably caused her death, that would only impress unbiased judges. I suppose the judges in question could not overcome the prejudice held by the general public, and accept incompetence of physicians and hospitals in regards to opioid addiction.

As a drug addict myself who took tons of narcotic medications, I knew and felt first-hand how these drugs negatively affected my clients, and the stigma and judgmental attitudes towards them. As a medical professional who evaluates patients with narcotic addictions, I could see and explain the harmful prescribing and addictive use, and adverse consequences. As an attorney, I had to combine my background to make my case and persuade the judge and jury. The defense often did not refute my allegations directly, and did not show particular medical and pharmacological knowledge to even offset my insightful and responsive offense.

Rather, the defense relied on the notion that the doctor was just doing his job, treating pain and responding to the patient's subjective complaints of it. The patient was at fault if they became addicted. The patient should show more control over their drug use. The patient lied if they did not need narcotics for pain, rather sought the narcotics to satisfy an addiction. The loss of control over her addictive drug use was not the responsibility of the doctor. The doctor bore no fault if they continued to give to and feed an addicted patient. The patient, not the doctor, should make decisions regarding the "legitimate need" to take narcotics for pain. Narcotic addiction did not exist if the doctor prescribed for pain, and if it did, it was the patient's choice to seek narcotics for pain.

I personally and professionally tried to explain all these critical thoughts and actions to the judge and jury. But I could not overcome the doctor, the stigma, or the judgmental attitudes towards addictions. Alcoholics and drug addicts are certainly not a protected class from discrimination. Rather, addicts and alcoholics are often discriminated against, regarded as criminals, while physicians can do no wrong when dealing with them. In treatment and recovery, we ask the addict/alcohol to be responsible for their actions, particularly, while they were addicted. An addict is not at fault for their addictive use. While they may have chosen to use an addicting drug, and accepted the physician's recommendation to take addicting narcotic medications, they are not at fault.

If the patient is responsible for accepting to use a narcotic medication for pain and becomes addicted, *why is the doctor not responsible for prescribing an addicting medication and addicting the patient?* Even if the doctor is trying to help relieve pain, they are not relieved of the responsibility to prescribe safely and responsibly. Whereas when the patient is seeking pain relief, they are not relieved of the responsibility for becoming addicted. Both are responsible, and neither is at fault if both exercise reasonable care, which includes the knowledge and skill in prescribing addicting medications. Since many doctors do not know how to safely prescribe addicting "pain killers," they are often subject to fault and liability.

I find that many doctors do not inform the patient that the medications are addicting as part of informed consent. A doctor is supposed tell the patient of the risks and benefits of treatment and alternative treatments, but many do not. Strangely and irresponsibly, the American Academy of Family Physicians published a position paper that it was a myth that narcotic medications were not addicting if prescribed for pain. The Mayo Clinic followed up with a similar statement that narcotics were not addicting if used for pain. I wonder how many patients would not have started on narcotic medications if they had been honestly and initially advised by their physicians of the potential and high probability to develop addiction.

Eventually, I ran into too many adverse court decisions due to the odd and oppressive plaintiff medical practice laws, as well as lack of money and experience, but mostly because of biased judges, courts, and public opinion. The State of Michigan passed tort reform years ago that limited the noneconomic damages with a cap, so that insurance companies could calculate in advance their exposure to liability. As many patients who became addicted due to physicians prescribing narcotics became disabled and lost employment, the damages to be recovered were dependent on limited pain and suffering unless proven that the physician prescribing caused unemployment. That is a tough job to accomplish.

I worked on a contingency basis and could not collect unless we won the case. I also supported the expenses and lost money if we did not collect money on the settlement or court award. Because I had to support myself working as a physician, working afternoons and evenings, driving long distances to patients in hospitals, eventually I ran out of gas. Ultimately, I could not afford to support myself, the children in college and a full caseload of medical practice cases without a flow of incoming revenue.

It was around this time, I began to look at my accumulation of debt, both personal and professional, as I took out student loans for thousands of dollars to pay for the girls' college costs, and credit cards. Also, I had taken out large amounts of money to pay for law school tuition expenses, and now for law practice. It all seemed crazy, and led to large amount of unsecured debt. I realized that I could not hope to support my mission to sue doctors and hospitals on debt alone. I knew I had to do something to stem my dependence on debt. I had visited and confronted this problem years ago, but had drifted away from my solution.

I now decided to return to a recovery program that had worked for me in the past. I had to confront an old nemesis, and to find a way to continue my missions. I picked up the phone and arranged to attend a Debtors Anonymous meeting in Ann Arbor. I had created a pretty complicated set of financial commitments without an income due to my debting addiction. What a predicament. Here I was, an accomplished and experienced psychiatrist and neurologist, a newly minted attorney, dedicated to a high risk medical malpractice, and had less than marginal economic means. Sounds like a familiar insanity I experienced elsewhere due to addictions.

"I think unconscious bias is one of the hardest things to get at."

—Ruth Bader Ginsburg

17

NEVER ENOUGH,
COMPULSIVE DEBTING

*"Solving a problem created by debt... by creating more
debt is a fool's errand."* —Olivier Sarkozy

When Kate was born in 1989, I knew I needed money for her college education., but I instinctively knew I had a problem with debt. I knew I could not afford to save for college for her with the way I spent and managed money. I had accumulated some $90,000 in credit card debt, was late on my house rental payments, and never had enough money for all my expenses. I even took my own pictures at my wedding reception. (Though I did hire a friend photographer for the actual wedding in the church). My biggest debt problem was unsecured debt. Basically, abstinence from compulsive debting involves not using or accumulating unsecured debt; unsecured debt is not backed up by collateral, and credit card debt is a common type.

I discussed my money issues with my AA sponsor who suggested I try Debtors Anonymous. DA is an organization patterned after AA, using the 12 Steps and tools, modified for debtors, and was based on the same spiritual solution to debting with money as with alcohol. I started attending meetings of DA, and noted an abrupt improvement in my debt and spending. Because in DA debting is viewed as an addiction problem, I fit right in. Just another addiction, this time to debt. Unsecured debt happens when I overspend or under earn. If I use unsecured debt such as credit card, I often overspend and curiously do not spend on my needs. Rather, I buy items that aren't necessities or cannot afford. In reality, I am compulsively spending, and as in compulsive alcohol or drug use, leading to adverse consequences; debt in its many forms.

I recognized that I could not continue accumulating large sums of debt while supporting my family then and in the future. I did not know why and how I debted and in such large amounts. I didn't think my addictions would extend to money, but I suppose, why shouldn't it? I had ignored money, thinking it and business were beneath me. My mother had always been very frugal and clever with money though never wealthy, never earning large sums. She left me partial-ownership of her house when she died. My father, on the other hand, made a good income but never managed it very well. He ran through businesses and spending on expensive homes and cars. He left me nothing when he died. What I found in DA was a sound road map on how to manage money, combined with a spiritual solution borrowed from the 12 Step program of Alcoholics Anonymous.

I learned in DA about the "Signs of Compulsive Debting," and how they applied to me. I was unclear about my financial situation. I did not know account balances, monthly expenses, loan interest rates, fees, fines, or contractual obligations. I probably kept most of my papers, but rarely examined or organized them. I just thought fees and interest rates were necessary and unavoidable, never understanding them, never paying them.

I frequently "borrowed" items such as books, pens,

or small amounts of money from friends and others, and failed to return them. My family was the object of my borrowing. I borrowed from my mother, wife, and father. My mother gave me money for school during early adulthood, with the understanding I would pay it back, which I never did. My father gave me cars, which I destroyed during my drinking days. And my wife used her equity from her home to support our buying new homes. I had little and contributed little. Worse yet, I had no understanding of my responsibilities with money.

To start, I had poor saving habits. Not planning for taxes, retirement, or other not-recurring but predictable items, and then feeling surprised when they come due. I had a, "Live for today, don't worry about tomorrow" attitude. Somehow, I tried to save through my work in 401k and 457 accounts. But my mounting debt obliterated most of any gains in savings. I sort of guessed at my taxes, and had to borrow money to pay income taxes due. I kind of held my breath and blocked out any thoughts of how to meet my taxes due, though I was fortunate enough to not ignore paying them. I did have one encounter with the Internal Revenue Service for taxes owed, and did not like the feeling that they could unilaterally claim my property or send me to prison. While I had many close calls, paying penalties, and interests, I thankfully avoided draconian measures by the IRS.

Also, I shopped compulsively. I was a master at compulsive spending, more likely to do with unsecured credit. I still tinker with being unable to pass up a "good deal"; making impulsive purchases; leaving price tags on clothes so they can be returned; not using items I'd purchased. I still have a closet full of shoes that I have never worn.

As a result of compulsive spending without a purpose, I accumulated clutter I am still trying to clear. I buy clothes, particularly, that I may not wear, or don't need. And I don't take an inventory of my existing clothes so I end up adding unneeded clothes to piles I already have or don't need. Not to mention, I can't find clothes I even use in all the clutter. I run out of storage space, and inexplicably keep adding expensive, useless clothing. That's the kind of addictive spending that leads to debting, when I use credit or money I need for something else. Whenever my spending exceeds my income, and I use unsecured credit, I debt. And if I use savings or money needed elsewhere, I deprive myself of resources.

I had difficulty in meeting basic financial or personal obligations, and/or an inordinate sense of accomplishment when such obligations are met. I was having trouble meeting my monthly mortgages, car payments, and other expenditures. In order to cover my compulsive debting, I turned to unsecured line of credit, or home equity loans, one was debting and the other led to compulsive debting. Whenever I made payments I felt like I had successfully climbed Mt. Everest. All the while, I was spiraling deeper in debt and in despair. I kept looking over a crevice, and sensing I would fall without a landing in sight. Similar to feelings I had when I was using drugs, I felt hopeless, helpless, and going nowhere fast. I always thought, *someday*! Someday I would make enough money to cover my spending. A thought I later learned I would never realize, as my compulsive spending and debt accumulation would always outpace my earnings.

I had a different feeling when buying things on credit than when paying cash, a feeling of being in the club, of being accepted, of being grown up. I remember when I got my very first credit card, an American Express card, it was then I had truly "arrived." I had always admired my father when he pulled out his American Express card. So special. My mother on the other hand, usually paid cash, and I looked down on her. Tightwad.

I had no conception of the difference between credit and cash. Particularly that cash was secured, and credit cards were not. Buying on credit gave me a feeling that I had an endless supply of money, and would never empty. A powerful, omnipotent feeling, intoxicated with credit. Whereas using cash left me with the terrified sense I would run out. I surrendered credit cards because I paid late, it was a huge hit on my credit score when I was late on mortgage payments. Another serious consequence of debting, similar to an addictive drinker losing their driver's license.

I lived in chaos and drama around money. Using one credit card to pay for another, bouncing checks, always having a financial crisis to contend with. Even after I stopped writing checks in a drunken black out, I still wrote checks without adequate funds, or knowing the amount of money in my account to cover the check. I was stunned when I ran out of money, despite the fact that I didn't keep track of it. Another way I perpetuated and inflated my debt was to use a credit card at 0% to pay off other credit cards. I would rack up thousands of dollars on 0% card to pay off higher interest cards. The problem was, I was not paying down credit card debt and took on new debt with 0% credit. And the 0% interest was for a limited time, after which the interest rate would escalate into usury levels.

Not to mention the amount of interest accumulating on unpaid balance. By paying the minimum each month someone could be trying to reduce and pay off balance for years, even a lifetime. It is frightening how much expense credit can incur by using it that way. I borrowed from Peter to pay Paul, and ended up deeper in debt. A continuous downward spiral into the same abyss I fell into during the addictive drug and alcohol use. I could not avoid accumulating high interest rates, and exponentially exploding balances. I ran faster and harder, and fell behind with every step and effort. Only darkness descended, light vanishing. Thank God for denial or I would have gone completely crazy, not just crazy.

I had a tendency to live on the edge. Living paycheck to paycheck, taking risks with health and car insurance coverage, writing checks hoping money will appear to cover them. That was me; I wrote checks with a wing and a prayer that money would appear out of thin air. I was living in steep denial regarding how my compulsive spending was making my life worse, not better, how I was living unsuccessfully paycheck to paycheck, and my whole world could come crashing down on me. Here I was, years into recovery from my alcoholism and drug addiction, and I was confronted by a new demon, compulsive spending and under earning.

I was never very good at money as I started to borrow in college to pay for my tuition, books, and drinking. I accumulated education debt just to keep me afloat and drunk. Inexplicably, that type of debting continued into my sober days, and was not affected by my recovery from drug and alcohol addictions. My intellect, common sense, and fear of debt did not lessen my risks to me and my family. On the one hand, I was able to cover some sins and debt with my power to earn as a physician, but my higher earnings just elevated the level of my debt accumulation. My total debt was ten times higher at an income of $100,000 than $10,000. Thus, greater earnings led to greater debt.

Despite doing well in mathematics and calculus as a student, I couldn't master these simple arithmetic calculations with my personal finance.

I had warranted inhibition and embarrassment in what should be a normal discussion of money. Even with my level of education, I had past use of secured and unsecured debt, and high utilization of money. I could not carry on nor understand discussions of money. I thought interest rates whether high or low were something you had to live with, pay no matter what, didn't really matter that much, 3% or 9% were still small numbers anyway, even if spread out over years. I would think nothing of refinancing a mortgage to lower the interest rate while drawing out thousands from equity to pay off other, unsecured debt. That might have been a reasonable strategy if I had not turned around and continued to compulsivly use unsecured debt. I was dealing in relatively large sums of money without clearly discussing or examining my moves.

I certainly had a large inhibition to learning about money, despite multiple undergraduate and graduate degrees, medical and law licenses, and board certifications. Believe it or not, no family, professional or friend, stepped forward to explain or confront me on my insanity with spending and money. Nor did they understand my spending. My mother would frequently retort when I complained about my lack of money, "You don't look like you spend very much." I later learned it is not only how much I spend, but *how* I spend. I would buy items I didn't need, use money I didn't have, neglect to spend on my needs, and deprive myself.

A dramatic example of my hitting bottom was when I started to take seriously to "not debt," I realized I did not have enough money to buy a bar of bath soap. So instead of reaching for a credit card, I scoured my house for change to buy soap. I had to resist the temptation to steal soap from my mother's house.

Working extra hours to earn money to pay creditors, I was using time inefficiently and taking jobs below my skill and education level. I certainly under earned when my employment ended at MSU. I continued to do some expert testimony and performed Independent Medical Evaluations. I also testified in criminal cases, something I liked doing. The pay was lucrative in instances, by the hour, and involved record reviews, interviewing the defendant, writing a report, and appearing in court on occasions. I performed a small number of IMEs where I evaluated claimants for short and long term disabilities from employment, and medical necessity for diagnostics and treatment. But I did no other work to speak of. I did not work in hospitals, or in an office practice.

As a result, I had to use credit cards, precious savings, and other sources of secured and unsecured credit. I actually existed for two to three years like this, until I decided to start work at a psychiatric hospital that was short lived. I didn't like full time clinical work, a long drive, and being so far away from my daughters, especially with the possibility of a looming re-abduction of them.

After I joined DA, I attended meetings on and off over the years, and started new meetings. My financial picture improved gradually. I mostly had academic jobs that paid below the market value of a psychiatrist in private practice. However, I saved as much as I could in pretax mutual funds, 401k accounts. I also bought real estate, a condo and a Lake Michigan residence. I picked properties that fulfilled location, location, location, and investments.

Debting is a common problem for many individuals

and businesses. Even the U.S. government is an example of spending money it does not have, and borrowing to pay bills it creates through entitlements. There is little correlation between spending laws passed and revenue generating through taxes. As a result, trillions of dollars of debt have accumulated on behalf of American citizens by government spending and debting. And there is no end in sight. There is no pay as you go or earn. Bankruptcy is the logical end.

It's magical how money appears when not debting is held fast, and a line is drawn in the sand. Shrouded denial and darkness surround the debtor, when the choice is using unsecured debt. As Sam Walton said, "Profits are made from expenses," which means reducing spending leads to savings, paradoxically. And debting erodes profit and savings.

Time and clutter become issues. Time devoted to generating income is mysteriously wasted when the focus is debting. Many debtors in DA under earn, taking jobs beneath them, working to chase debt that is a never-ending defeat. Some don't work at all, becoming destitute and bankrupt. Clutter accumulates when spending is not directed on needs, rather compulsive spending that is not calculated to satisfy needs. Closets become full of clothes with price tags not worn, excessive houses purchased, and cars leased that made no economic sense, met no logical needs. Just a trail of debt remains, and tension, anxiety, and desperation on how needs will be met and paid for.

I borrowed for law school tuition and money to live on because the loans were available. I also borrowed heavily for the girls' tuition at the University of Michigan for their undergraduate years. There were no restrictions to borrow large sums for parents. The law school and U-M were only too happy to push these loans as it provided more money to them to charge for increased tuition. The schools pro-moted more student debt (unsecured) and student debtors who borrowed for much more than school needs, e.g. homes, new cars, clothes, with no guarantee or means to pay the loans back. The easily available loan money caused schools to increase their expenses and tuition for the stu-dents, since they knew the students could get unsecured loan money without much restriction or requirement. The net effect is to make education more expensive and univer-sities to become bloated and inefficient.

I now have one large educational loan from law school left. I do not debt one day at a time. I live abundantly and prosperously. I still support my children and girlfriend. I apply the program to my life on a daily basis. I am grateful for the Business Debtors Anonymous (BDA) program and attend meetings weekly. I rigorously work the steps and apply the tools to my business and personal lives.

I had graduated from law school and passed the state bar, and become a licensed attorney. I wanted to live out my mission, and started chasing windmills like Don Quixote. I started a law practice in a Quixote fashion with similar outcomes, badly beaten and overcome. As a true debtor, I began a type of law practice, plaintiff medical malpractice, based on contingency work, which would re-quire expenditures without revenue in most cases. A natural set up for further debting.

Here I was, trying to carry out a mission from God to help the addicted, while immersed in my own debt addic-tion. Just as Don Quixote, I did not imagine reality correctly; construing reality was convenient for me. Adding a large dose of grandiosity that propelled me forward as the fic-tional knights, believing that justice and being in the right, would magically make money appear to support my worthy causes. This magical thinking disguised my actual reality, as I just dug myself deeper into debt. I don't want to forget my self-righteousness, that I was right, and right no matter what. Whoever disagreed with me was wrong and a phony.

Anyway, I racked up debt that could only be erased if I made money in a settlement or trial verdict in cases. In the meantime, I kept becoming deeper in debt. During one of my pressure relief group meetings, a fellow recovering debtor asked, "When are you going to stop the bleeding?" It had become evident that I could not win these cases against the resources of insurance companies, the prejudice of the courts, and the extremely pro defense of doctors among jurists. So I began my descent and withdrawal from filing lawsuits and stepped up my income from various forms of medical practice litigation. I gave up my dream from law school to change bias and prejudice against addicts to hold doctors responsible, to change medical education and care in addictions.

I had learned in DA how to earn, and earn efficiently. My income gradually escalated, and I paid off large amounts of debt belonging to educational loans. I had accumulated education debt from my law school and the girls' college education. The law school and university were only too happy to loan me money. The more loans they could force students and parents to take out, the higher tuition amounts they could charge to inflate their operating budget. In a sense, the college and University could raise tuition and other expenses, eg. housing, etc, when students and parents took out greater amounts of debt in form of loans. Kind of like extortion, or exploitation at least.

Another symptom of my debting was that I had an unwillingness to care for and value myself. Living in self-imposed deprivation; denying my basic needs in order to pay my creditors. I looked pretty good on the outside but on the inside I was desperately trying to ward off creditors and consequences of debt. I was a doctor and a lawyer, yet I had to borrow to stay afloat. I was making business and financial decisions that only worsened my bottom line. When I had to search for "change," to buy a bar of soap and avoid debting to do it, I realized how deprived I had become. I could not afford the cars and homes I bought on credit, although secured, and had to use credit cards to pay the bills.

In turn, I had become a slave to my creditors. So the pile of debt was the first set of obligations or sentencing I worked on. I can remember I owed $30,000 on one credit card, and several others with similarly large amounts. Fortunately, the education debt was not due, but it was accumulating debt at 7% on mounting balances. I could not or would not value myself over my debt. Debt was my supreme preoccupation. I could not afford, except with further debt, anything else. I was living on the edge of the precipice, dangling hopelessly, looking down on another abyss from addiction. I experienced the same intoxication with debt and the helplessness, as I did with alcohol and drugs. I deprived myself with debt in similar ways I did with alcohol and drugs.

I had a feeling that someone would take care of me if necessary, so that I wouldn't really get into serious financial trouble; that there would always be someone I could turn to. When growing up, it was my mother who would get me out of financial trouble. She would always come up with money somehow. As I drank my way through college and medical school, I relied on her to send some money when I was in a jam, which was pretty often. My father chipped in with a car now and then. I was living pretty frugally, wearing only a few washable shirts and pants, living in a rental house with roommates or a girlfriend. My then girlfriend actually even supported me. So I had another to turn to for money.

I didn't really start to accumulate debt until I made money, but I lived in quasi deprivation while in school and residencies. When my mother refused to give me more money, ran out of girlfriends to support me, and got a job to get big credit, that's when I really started to get into serious financial trouble. I carried the conviction with me that someday I would make so much money I would pay off all the debt, and would never have to worry about money. Well, as you know I never reached that point, and probably never will in my lifetime.

I actively use the tools of Debtors Anonymous in my recovery. These tools are derived from common sense. They are sound financial practices applied to a 12 Step spiritual recovery program. Recovery from compulsive debting begins when we stop incurring new, unsecured debt, one day at a time, as it did for me. (Unsecured debt is any debt that is not backed up by some form of collateral, such as a house or other asset). We attain a daily reprieve from compulsive debting by practicing the 12 Steps and by using the DA Tools.

When I abstain from incurring unsecured debt one day at a time, I achieve and maintain abstinence from compulsive debt just as I do when I abstain from alcohol in maintaining my abstinence. I achieve solvency in DA when my assets exceed my liabilities, just as defined in other areas of finance. Some of us, myself included, were solvent, having more assets than liabilities but having unsecured debt in large amounts, as in my case. Some of us are bankrupt. I was fortunate not to be in that state but I easily could have if I had maintained my course of compulsive debting. Just as in my recovery in AA, I had to take actions, and those right actions led to right thinking, and success in my dealings with money and debt. I am here to tell you by using the 12 Tools of Debtors Anonymous and working the 12 Steps, I not only stopped debting but worked my way out of debt, and into abundance and prosperity. While the feelings of never having enough still haunt me, I have a positive balance, do not debt one day at a time, and have an optimistic outlook on my financial life, though not as wealthy as I would like, nor as secure as I want to be. However, in the final analysis how secure can anyone be? Assets can dissolve at any time, stock or real estate market can crash, banks can go bankrupt, the dollar can lose its value, and I can forfeit my savings, perhaps overnight.

Nonetheless these are the outcomes I cannot control. God grant me the serenity to accept the things I cannot change, like the markets, world, and the courage to change the things I can, such as my debting and recovery, and the wisdom to know the difference. I require a constant vigilance to spend my attention and efforts on certain tools and the 12 steps.

I attend meetings at which I share my experience, strength, and hope with others. Unless I give to newcomers what we have received from DA, I cannot keep it out. I attend weekly meetings, mostly over the phone in conference calls, though I have attended in person meetings, actually even started up new meetings. These days I prefer meetings in the morning on the phone, and avoid the evening in person meetings. I also avoid contentious personal interactions to focus on principles and not personalities.

Meetings typically last 30 minutes to an hour, have a structure, timed shares, and prepared readings. We repeat favorite prayers with references to God or a Creator, but in a spiritual, not religious way. During the meeting we are careful to follow the structure to insure order for everyone's participation. We are not confrontative, critical, or judgmental. Rather compassionate, understanding, and loving as much as possible with each other. We are human, emotional creatures who are successful in varying degrees in our efforts.

I maintain records of my daily income and expenses, records of my savings, and of the retirement of any portions of my outstanding debts. This is common sense, a practical tool that not many of us used in our chaotic days of denial and confusion. I did not know when and what bills were due back then. I did not plan for taxes or major expenses to meet. I lacked clarity around basic accounting, could not balance my accounts until I started using the Quicken program. It was pretty easy to miss due dates, and rack up credit, not knowing.

I record my numbers mostly in Quicken so I can generate reports that show me how much and from where I earned income, and spent money. I experienced an amazing difference in my spending, and eventually my income by knowing what came in and went out. Now I am motivated, like a business, to earn to meet my expenses by keeping track of the balance. I know these are basic tools that individuals and businesses use, but they are frequently near absent in compulsive debtors.

I found it essential to my recovery to have a sponsor and to be a sponsor. A sponsor is a recovering debtor who guides us through the 12 Steps and shares his or her own experience, strength, and recovery. I still don't know exactly why this works but sponsorship is very helpful. Direct feedback in addition to indirect feedback from meetings is invaluable. Also, many of the steps are designed to be shared with another individual, to avoid staying in the dark due to denial or lack of action. A sponsor is a source of clarity that is hard to duplicate in meetings. Also, sponsors are very helpful on a personal level in working the 4th and 5th Steps.

After I had gained some familiarity with the DA program, I organized Pressure Relief Groups (PRGs) and Pressure Relief Meetings consisting of myself and two other recovering debtors who had not incurred unsecured debt for at least 90 days and who had a longer history in the program. The group meets in a series of Pressure Relief Meetings to review my financial situation. These meetings typically result in the formulation of a spending plan and an action plan. You might consider this strategic planning that businesses undertake to plan missions, targets, expenses, and profits.

The Pressure Relief Groups are intended to ease pressure through group examination, not increase it. Typically, the debtor prepares with a record of income and expenses, assets, liabilities, visions, goals, and importantly pressure points. Pressure points may be for the beginner how to deal with mountains of debt, or for the more advanced what are their visions and goals. The Group examines sources of pressure for debting through spending and earnings, and hard to achieve realizations of visions, such as starting or improving a business, paying for a car, mortgage, college education, or just plain digging out of debt and staying out of debt. The ultimate goal for our recovery is to live abundantly and prosperously.

Per DA tools, I developed a spending plan putting my needs first that gives me clarity and balance in my spending. It includes categories for income, spending, debt payment, and savings (to help me build cash reserves, however humble). The income plan helps me focus on increasing my income. The debt payment category guides me in making realistic payment arrangements without depriving myself. Savings can include prudent reserves, retirement, and special purchases. Believe it or not, a determined, recorded, and clear spending plan, is missing in most debtors. Many debtors have little clarity regarding income and expenses, as they try to avoid the bad news. In doing so, they compound the debting and deprivation.

Developing a spending plan like the other tools require discipline, but the difference between the old days and the new days for me, is that there is a recovery based on group support, tools, and spiritual power through the 12 Steps of DA. Discipline in DA is a "Good Orderly Direction" for abundance and prosperity, and not self-imposed punishment, atonement or penance. By taking actions, I, as a debtor, spring into new dimensions where I am doing things that I could not do previously.

With the help of our Pressure Relief Group, I developed a list of specific actions in a plan for resolving my debts, improving my financial situation, and achieving my goals without incurring unsecured debt. The plan includes specific actions for my visions, spending and income plans, special purchases, and any other. Because I am self-employed, have a business in medicine and law, and have a personal financial life, I keep separate accounts for each and make transfers between accounts. I have different plans for business from personal, and keep spending records and expenses for each.

An action plan is like directions in a road map or GPS to guide me. DA like AA is an action program, and I attain a daily reprieve from compulsive debting by practicing the 12 Steps and using these tools. DA is based on the 12 Steps, and utilizes similar spiritual solutions to our compulsive debting problems. As you can see, the tools are common sense business practices that are universally used, and incorporated into the recovery model. The idea is to take actions to generate spiritual growth to grow financially, in abundance and prosperity.

I maintain frequent contact with other DA members through phone, email, and other forms of communication. I make a point of talking to other DA members before and after taking difficult steps in our recovery. This practice is called bookending, and is an invaluable tool to confer with others regarding financial and other actions. Again, it's a common sense approach.

I study the literature of Debtors Anonymous and of Alcoholics Anonymous to strengthen my understanding of compulsive disease and of recovery from compulsive debting. Compulsive debting and compulsive alcohol and drug use are very similar in that both are addictions. The root problem of both is addiction, and solutions are actions and spirituality. The word debt can be substituted for alcohol and drugs in the *Big Book of Alcoholics Anonymous* without losing any meaning, and is instructive in either compulsive debting or drug use.

I maintain awareness of the danger of compulsive debt by taking note of bank, loan companies, as well as credit card advertising, and their effects on us. I also remain aware of my personal finances in order to avoid vagueness, which can lead to compulsive debting or spending. As a result, I have learned much about business and finance. I read the business/money sections of the newspaper, subscribe to the *Wall State Journal, Kiplinger Reports, Fortune Magazine*, and other leading publications.

Maintaining clarity for my spending and income, is

key as ambiguity leads to compulsive debting. I also do not really know what my needs are if I am not clear, and I want to avoid clutter which disguises my needs with wants. I have had closets filled with clothes and shoes I bought compulsively, and I also clutter by not turning over shirts and pants, which I keep forever. I hold onto them for reasons only a debtor would know.

I attend DA business meetings that are held monthly. For one, I had long harbored feelings that "business" was not a part of my life but for others more qualified. Actually, I was arrogant that business was beneath me, and that I was too good for it. Yet participation in running our own program teaches us how our organization operates and also helps us to become responsible for our own recovery. Attending business meetings takes ultimate patience and restraint, as I know what is good for me, and for you. I can't understand why you won't do what I say.

I perform service at various levels: personal, meeting, and intergroup. Service is vital to my recovery. Only through service can I give to others what so generously has been given to me. Service for me takes several forms, such as attending and leading meetings, sitting in on PRGs, bookending with another DA member, keeping time for shares during the meeting, doing readings from DA literature. In doing service, I stay connected to the DA program, and offer to others what has helped me. Service is a spiritual exercise, and by "giving it away, I can keep," and grow in my recovery by helping others. Helping others has been a cornerstone in my spiritual development, which is focused on and centered in very practical results.

Just as I develop and maintain my desire not to drink by working with other alcoholics, I do the same to maintain and develop my desire not to debt one day at a time by working with debtors. As it says in the *Big Book of Alcoholics Anonymous*, "Practical experience shows that nothing will so much insure immunity from drinking as intensive work with other alcoholics." The same applies to my experience in Debtors Anonymous, that working with others will ensure immunity from compulsive debting.

In DA, we practice anonymity, which allows me freedom of expression by assuring us that what we say at meetings or to other DA members at any time will not be repeated. Anonymity is key also to my spiritual development, without which I would expose myself to problems with ego and grandiosity. Anonymity helps me practice humility.

Also, revealing in a public manner that I am recovering from compulsive debting may attract stigma and negative consequences as with alcoholism. Keeping my head down is really important in maintaining recovery, and recovery is necessary for me to not compulsively debt. In DA, "In order to lead normal, happy and useful lives, we try to practice to the best of our ability certain principles in all our daily affairs."

I had arrived at a crossroad. One road, a soft road, lures me on to further despair, illness, ruin, and in some cases, mental institutions, prison or suicide. The other road, a more challenging road, leads to self-respect, solvency, healing, and personal fulfillment. I decided to take the first difficult step onto the more solid road now, and continued to do so to abundance and prosperity.

I'll be back in the high life again
All the eyes that watched me once will smile and take me in

—"Back in the High Life Again" Steve Winwood

18

SEX AND FOOD ADDICTIONS

"He that will not apply new remedies
must expect new evils." —Francis Bacon

I cannot tell the truth about my sex life without embarrassment. I can talk about my drinking and drug use without problems, even debting and spending without being overly self-conscious. But my sex life is very hard to talk to you about, and even harder to describe my feelings and sexual acts. I certainly do not want to embarrass women I had sexual encounters with, and enjoyed every one I had sex with. Unlike my drinking I recall pleasure and excitement, and have good memories about my erotic experiences. But I still had problems due to my addiction to sex, preoccupation with sex experiences with women, compulsive sex acts with and without women present, and a pattern of continuous relapse to sexual behaviors. Similar to compulsive drinking and debting, I had developed a maladaptive pattern of sexuality that interfered with my relationships, psychological well being, and led ultimately to a life of isolation from women altogether.

Because sex addiction is akin to other forms of addictions, it is often found in alcoholics and drug addicts, and even debtors. I find considerable connections between debting, sex, drinking, all with addictive behaviors. I can see preoccupation, compulsive use, and relapse with sex, drinking, drugging, and debt. There are areas in the brain that are responsible for these addictions, namely, the midbrain and limbic structure in the phylogenetically old parts of the brain or instincts. Instinctive or unconscious drives were found in animals way back, probably billions of years ago. These are the basis for survival, such as reproduction, hunger, protection, thirst, that depend on reward systems for continued expression.

From dopamine neurons in the midbrain, the mesolimbic pathway projects to limbic lobe forward in the brain to the nucleus accumbens. The mesolimbic pathway is responsible for reward behaviors; we feel pleasure when we engage in sexual activity or even when thinking about it. Similarly, we feel pleasure with certain addicting drugs, alcohol, and even spending money. Common to all these sensations is excitement; sex ignites excitement that is sometimes extreme, and drugs, spending, and buying items can do the same. I can still think of nude women and feel good. I would imagine the same is true of women, thinking of men and getting excited.

What happens in these addictions is that these drives states become associated with and entrained by sex, drugs, money, and yes, even rock and roll. A strong connection develops between the reward centers in the brain and sex, drugs, money, and rock and roll, but the connection eventually becomes short circuited and out of control, and then not so pleasurable. Normally, I have some control over my drives to some extent, but not completely. These drive states are all powerful and hard to resist, as they are responsible for survival.

When the pursuit of sex, drugs, or money becomes out of control, bad things and adverse consequences happen. Too much of anything, even good things cause problems. People are involved in sex acts and many taboos, customs and practices, govern sexual behaviors and interactions. So much so that we find it hard to talk about sex, and even practice it sometimes.

If we start to satisfy our sex drive indiscriminately whenever and however we will it, you can see how much trouble a person, like myself, can cause themselves and others. Laws regarding sexual activity are so strict, we cannot even buy it. And morals and ethics don't allow us to engage with different partners, and proscribe we do it with only one partner if in a relationship. Our superego punishes us and we get complaints if we want just sexual gratification without the emotional attachments and personal obligations.

As with other forms of addiction in the extreme, sexual addiction, which is also called sexual dependency, hypersexuality, nymphomania (females), satyriasis (males), is compulsive sexual behavior and sexual compulsivity, and refers to the phenomenon in which people cannot manage their sexual behavior. I can be obsessed with sexual thoughts, thoughts which interfere with my ability to work properly, have relationships, and go about my daily activities.

Many say that sexual addiction is a form of obsessive-compulsive behavior. A person with sexual addiction is obsessed with sex, or has an abnormally intense sex drive. My life at times was dominated with sex and the thought of sex, so much so that other activities and interactions became seriously affected. It is not uncommon for someone with sexual addiction to rationalize and justify their behavior and thought patterns. People with a sex addiction may deny there is a problem, as I did.

There is a strong link between sexual addiction and risk-taking. Even though the risk of danger is clear, addicts may take risks regardless of the potential consequences, even if this means possible health problems (sexually transmitted diseases), fertility risks or emotional consequences. As a sex addict I may initially be involved in a healthy and enjoyable sexual situation that eventually develops into an obsession. Or my obsession with sex develops into a relationship that later fails outside of the sexual excitement. Fantasies and sometimes actual acts may be well outside the radar of most people's idea of what is sexually acceptable behavior.

I guess everyone has a different idea when it comes to sex. Sex is very funny thing. We think of sex very often I think, it is on our minds whenever we meet someone, yet hardly ever talk about it and usually do not act on our sexual impulses. I would be surprised if we didn't size up sex in most people we encounter. Sex is a very powerful drive in our lives, one way or the other.

I felt a of lack of control in my sexual addiction, a feeling that I was unable to resist impulses to engage in sexual acts. I found myself engaging in sexual behaviors for much longer than they had intended, and to a much greater extent. There have been several attempts to stop, reduce, or control behaviors. I spent a great deal of time obtaining sex, being sexual, or recovering from a sexual experience. I gave up social, work-related or recreational activities because of my sexual addiction. If our sexual aggression becomes too extreme, we may forcefully overcome to satisfy our sexual desires. Or expose ourselves to unwanted outcomes, pregnancy, diseases, conflicts in relationships, legal problems.

I told you about my sexual experiences during my

drinking and in my early recovery. I certainly experienced high levels of pleasure and excitement. I don't think I necessarily picked out a woman and said to myself, "I want to have sex with her, she excites me." Most of the time it just happened. I had many encounters without use of contraceptives or protections from disease, a sign of my overall problem. I also had many encounters with women for only one episode, or a short-term relationship that did not last for very long. I moved from one intimate, sexual encounter to another, enjoying vivid memories of my sensual experience.

I could perform for long periods and experimented with different erotic positions. Excitement and pleasure were my goals, but I wanted my partners to experience similar sensations. It was not enough for me to feel good during the sexual acts, it was just as important for my partner to enjoy along with me.

I recall one difficult relationship, where we frequently argued over just about everything except our sex. She would imply I was not good for much except, "making love." More than one woman gave me that vote of confidence. However, in one relationship, we would end long, loud arguments with a long, sensuous, intercourse. Even with some intimacy. I had sincere feelings towards some of my sexual encounters, others were objects of mutual pleasure. However, some women accused me of being a "sex addict" with my focus on the sex, and they even noted my glazed look during the intercourse.

I had to find the women I was with to be attractive to me in order to stimulate my sexual desires. I've admitted before, I was particularly excited by blondes, but it really didn't matter too much if they were beautiful. I obviously had some control, as I did not have sex with every attractive woman around! I can say that I never forced myself on anyone, though I may have been too persistent at times. I can also say the opposite was true, that women pursued me, and lured or pressed me, for sexual pleasure. I was particularly adept at one-night stands where the mutual goal was a brief sexual encounter, with no strings attached, and no recurrent sex or return encounters. Believe or not, I remember those as well.

As addicts progress in their recovery from alcohol and drug addiction, and their sex addiction emerges even more obviously, they may begin the regular practice of masturbation, usually alone. At first, it was just photos, videos, and magazines. Later, the Internet brought a whole new dimension to my sexual activity. Now one could instantly access photos, and especially, videos of sexuality. I think the Internet's sexual graphics have entrapped many males particularly, young and old. A common problem among young men is compulsive masturbation while watching "pornography."

I won't attempt to define pornography beyond the Supreme Court's holding, "You will know it when you see it." Like alcohol or money, I don't think in and by themselves they are bad or evil in intent. It's what they do to you. What is wrong with looking at a nude body? Nothing I can think of. What is wrong with masturbation? A relatively normal male or female sexual activity, just like drinking or spending money. But when that activity assumes a preoccupation, compulsive use and continued pattern of return or relapse, then the addiction sets in and adverse consequences ensue, with its doom, ruin, and destruction of mind, body, and soul.

What young men report, and what I experienced, was compulsive masturbation while watching Internet videos of sexuality, that then precluded desire and prevented performance in sexual relations with an intimate partner; the intimate partner that you were in a committed relationship with. Not only desire for sexual contact was missing with an otherwise attractive partner, but absent was the ability to initiate and maintain an erection, and ultimately achieve ejaculation and release. Such a stunning experience.

Unfortunately, compulsive masturbation interferes with mature relationships, particularly, as I grew older, one consequence of pornography being younger women became increasingly attractive to me. Many young men inexplicably could not find sex of interest in their girlfriends, and would continue to masturbate compulsively to strange women, sex scenes, and impersonal characters and situations.

I did certain things regarding my sex behaviors that I did in my drinking and debting days. I lied frequently about using the Internet, viewing nudes in published matter, and would "cheat" on my partner with my use of the Internet to view nude women instead of her. Imagine how that made her feel. I was flirting frequently with other women, gawking at them, seemingly more interested in younger women than her. I developed extreme confidence in my sexual prowess; grandiose in thinking I could excite every woman. I flirted all the time, sizing up and giving the eye and undressing every woman I saw in mind. Even transmitting to her sexual energy and desire I felt when looking at her, purely sexual. I had nothing in the way of a deep emotional cathexis, but I did feel a strong sexual desire and connection without commitments. When I was confronted, I did a two-step and tried to manipulate myself out of the jam I was in. I would do anything to get her off my back, to leave me alone, and not pressure me on my addiction and its effects on her.

There is much more help available today compared to even just a few years ago. Sex Addicts Anonymous (SAA) is a 12 Step program for sex addicts. The group was founded in 1977, by men who sought a greater sense of anonymity in other 12 Step sex addiction programs. SAA says it is a safe place for heterosexuals, homosexuals, and bisexuals who wish to treat their addictive sexual behaviors. A growing number of SAA groups initially give the enquirer a questionnaire, which is used to determine whether a prospective member is likely to be a sex addict. An SAA member creates their own definition of sexual sobriety, a personalized list of compulsive sexual behaviors from which they will abstain. SAA encourages members to respect each other's definition of sobriety.

While I don't attend SAA meetings, I do read a daily reflection book, called *Answers in the Heart*. And I apply the 12 Steps to my sex addiction. I can't say I am always completely abstinent from self-stimulating sexual episodes, but I certainly have more control and greater abstinent periods from compulsive masturbation and pornography. I certainly still notice women who wear revealing clothes, and I look, trying not to stare.

My daily reflection book focuses on the social isolation and emotional bankruptcy sex addicts experience. I have experienced that first hand. I spend my time with myself, have difficulty forming relationships with women, mostly fantasizing about women sexually. I do get an emotional charge that is returned by women, but it is based on sexual energy and not personal connections, or empathy.

However, I am able to connect in a relationship now to the best of my ability. Though not perfect, I am able to confine my emotional energy, and a good deal of my sexual energy to one relationship. I did not have extra sexual affairs or encounters outside relationships for the most part, but I was not perfect there either. Just as with my other addictions, I must apply the 12 Steps and tools to abstain from drugs, alcohol, debting, sex, and yet another addiction, food...

I am a compulsive overeater, or have a food addiction. I know that ultimately because I am overweight, and have been for a good deal of my adult life. I was not overweight as a child and adolescent, but obesity does run in my family. Remember, my father weighed over 300 lbs. basically because he ate too much, and likely ate compulsively. I always thought it was strange that I did not see him overeat, but he was always overweight. He preached moderation, but could not find it in his own appetite, or use of alcohol, or spending. He remarked how much I ate, but I did that in front of everyone. He did not. He was deflecting his problems on to me.

I struggle to keep my weight down, and don't eat that much, at least to me. But I do exhibit certain behaviors that would classify me as a compulsive overeater. I eat beyond my hunger points, my appetite is greater than my hunger, and I do not have an appetite that regulates the amount of food I eat. I typically feel an uncontrolled drive to consume food.

I am embarrassed about my weight and how my clothes don't fit. My stomach is protruding and my belt is tight. I feel uncomfortable and heavy, even now. My Body Mass Index (BMI) is over the recommended 25, just short of the obese range over 30. I am uncertain how predictive the BMI is for health, but it does show I am overweight. I barely eat, according to some people, but I do snack. I cannot for the life of me lose weight as much as I would like to. I don't have any metabolic abnormities except genes for obesity. I stay just under the fasting blood sugar limits for chemical Diabetes Mellitus, which also runs in my family.

I can control my weight the best when I my count caloric intake, and approximate expenditures. As I grow older my caloric requirements decrease. Just how much my genetic contribution of obesity affects my weight, caloric intake, and caloric requirements is not clear to me. I do have a persistent desire to lose weight and live at a lower weight.

I don't really go on eating binges per say, but the amount of food I eat varies. Some meals are lower in calories and I eat less. I can eat sensibly and then lose control. People would say I eat a healthy diet. I do however, over indulge when I dine in restaurants. And I feel guilty, as if I have let myself down if I overeat. The net result for me is that I eat too much for my caloric requirements. Checking myself on the scale can be a discouraging practice as my weight can fluctuate widely with fluid intake and retention. It can vary as much as 6-8 lbs. over a couple of days due to water retention and loss.

In simple terms, in order for me to maintain a certain weight, my caloric intake must match my caloric expenditures for no net gain or loss. If I want to lose weight, I must use more calories than I take in. A rule of thumb with exceptions is that 3500 calories equal a pound in weight. But we burn calories from muscle as well as fat as we lose weight. The more fat we have to lose, the more calories come from fat, and less from muscle. The faster we lose weight, the more likely we are to lose muscle mass. It's the fat we want gone, so gradual weight loss is better to lose fat. Most of us want to keep our muscle physique, but lose the frumpy appearances.

Obesity is common, serious, and costly. More than

one-third (36.5%) of U.S. adults are obese. Obesity-related conditions include heart disease, stroke, Type 2 diabetes, and certain types of cancer; some of the leading causes of preventable death. The estimated annual medical cost of obesity in the U.S. was $147 billion in 2008; the medical costs for people who are obese were $1,429 higher than those of normal weight.

These statistics do not measure the low self-esteem, social impairment, low energy, motivation, or personal estrangement that obese and overweight people experience daily. I know in my case, I have much more confidence when I am less heavy. I am also conscious of the medical risks I incur with being overweight and fight hard to keep my weight down, to look and feel better, to stay alive, healthier and longer.

My main problem I believe, with eating and weight, is that my appetite, not hunger, is set higher than my caloric requirements to maintain a lower weight. In other words, my appetite tells me I must maintain a "fat" weight, so my drive to eat is set higher than my ideal BMI. In a sense, my eating is out of control for my healthy weight. I am set at a higher weight than my health permits. Appetite and hunger are part of those same ancient drive states, along with thirst, sex, reproduction, that are connected to the reward system.

When I start to eat, I stimulate an uncontrolled drive state, and I want to eat more. If I don't eat, it is easier to control my appetite, as I did not stimulate my drive to eat. Which is why restrictive diets are sometimes preferred and work better than a reduction in daily calories. The problem is, when I resume eating, I provoke that same drive state and am off to the races again.

Unfortunately, the consequences for higher drive

states are things like obesity, sex addiction, intoxication, and all the complex problems associated with out of control instincts. The judgmental attitudes and morality enter because we should be able to control our appetites or drive states. When we don't, we are judged morally inept and bad. Our behaviors in regards to food, sex, drugs, are judged as unethical. I deserve the negative consequences of my excessive actions, even though I am not willful or intentional, but just having difficulties managing hard to control instinctive drives. Remember drive states are useful, ensure survival, and bring a measure of satisfaction to our daily living. Without reward for these instinctive behaviors, I would not survive.

In a sense, I am a victim of these addictive diseases. I did not set my level or strength of my drive states. Contrary to popular belief, I do not "will" my instinctive drives, as they come naturally, and I must respond to them. If I had a choice, I would reset my drive states to a lower level. Whatever pleasure I get from these drives is outweighed by the negative consequences. I am not happy fat, estranged from intimate relationship, excessively preoccupied sexually with women, intoxicated, impaired, depressed, and anxious from drugs and alcohol.

Although I do not practice per say the Overeaters Anonymous' 12 Step program of recovery from compulsive overeating, I developed my own plan for eating. I try to eat mostly healthy foods, such as salads, vegetable, fresh fruit, chicken, and fish, practically eliminating red meat. I do fall down by eating French fries and potato chips. I eat chocolates, and other licorice for dessert at times. I count calories, both what I eat and exercise, to try to keep weight gain down and live healthier and longer.

A plan of eating helps me abstain from compulsive

eating, and to deal with the physical aspects of our disease and achieve physical recovery. I also incorporate into my daily devotions a book that provides me with messages about overeating and the spiritual aspects of recovery.

Overeating is a physical, mental, and spiritual disease as is debting, alcoholism, and drug addiction, and I use a plan of action and spiritual source of power to help control my overeating and its consequences. I use the 12 Steps of Overeaters Anonymous in my daily life, as I do the 12 Steps of AA, NA, and DA. Because they are so similar I can use the same spiritual approach.

I am not at my desired weight nor do I think at my healthy weight. But I am not objectionably heavy and not yet unhealthy. I work out regularly, swimming, and walking on a regular basis, and have no outstanding medical conditions nor psychiatric concerns for that matter. I read daily meditation books on compulsive sex and eating, and work with my higher power to improve both addictions. I try hard meet my expectations but do not lose hope if I relapse or fail. I am not keeping score, not in contest. I am trying to do God's will in all my affairs, particularly addictions.

Sex, drugs, rock, roll
Sex, drugs, rock, roll

—"Sex & Drugs & Rock & Roll"
Ian Dury & the Blockheads

19

INSANITY

*"Insanity: doing the same thing over and over again
and expecting different results."* —Albert Einstein

My mind could bear plenty of reality, but not too much consistent gloom. When I woke up that night and went downstairs into the basement to try to take my life, I had little prior thoughts of suicide. I did have plenty of gloom and doom with crippling and demoralizing depression. I had become hopeless and helpless in my struggles with narcotic addictions. It was as if a switch went off in my mind to finally end this agony. My mind directed me to terminate my hapless condition. I instinctively knew what to do to kill myself. Suicide is killing by self, whether intentionally or unintentionally. In my case, I never intentionally wanted to die; my near death was a consequence of my out of control drug addiction. I involuntarily tried to off myself while under the influence of a compulsion to destroy myself.

Here I am, a recovering drug addict and alcoholic, my main purpose in my recovery is to carry the message. Step 12 states, "Having had a spiritual awakening as result of these steps, we tried to carry this message to alcoholics (drug addicts), and to practice these principles in all our affairs." However, I extended my personal recovery to my professional work. I understand that is not necessary recovery work, but I personally react in my professional work with alcoholics and drug addicts.

As you can see, there is no shortage of patients suffering from addictive diseases. In fact, an overabundance of patients with addictions, many caused by physicians who prescribe addicting medications unwittingly or carelessly, do so with little skill and knowledge of addictive diseases. They receive something like six hours education on addictions in medical schools and not much more in residency training. Add that to doctors' typical arrogant and negative attitudes towards addicted patients, and you have mixture of death, disability, and destruction. Doctors' prescribing of addicting medications leads to further medication induced psychiatric and medical conditions and diseases. Not to mention the enormous costs for unnecessary and fraudulent medical care.

Opioids, alcohol, stimulants, and other addicting drugs induce depression through their intoxicating effects. Narcotic and opioid drugs are classified as depressants, as is alcohol. Stimulants, through intoxicating effects, also produce depression. Depression has many causes, maybe hundreds, or thousands of causes, and is really a symptom or syndrome for other causes. In my case, narcotics, sedatives, and alcohol were the culprits and drug addiction was the root of it.

Why I continued to use these depressing and lethal drugs is the mystery of addiction. I was defenseless against the next pill, and in my case, the next bottle of pills, and the anguish that followed. Death was my solution. My mind could not tolerate the hopeless compulsion, as I was under the control and influence of toxic drugs. I felt as though I was being whipped and dragged, powerless to defend myself. What was left? Extermination? Just as I had little conscious control of my drug use, I had little conscious control of my self-inflicted death.

Suicide is the 10th leading cause of death in the U.S., and accounts for 34,000 deaths per year. An even greater number of people attempt suicide, as many as 5% of adults have attempted suicide. Alcohol and drugs are leading contributors to and are strongly related to suicide. Alcohol and drugs induce psychiatric symptoms and in that sense, cause mental illness. Someone with drug and alcohol addictions is six times more likely than someone without to make a suicide attempt in their lifetime. Men with drug and alcohol addiction are 2.3 times more likely to die by suicide than those without. Among women, drug and alcohol addiction increases the risk of suicide by 6.5 fold. Past history of suicide attempts is a strong risk factor for suicide. Depressed mood from drugs and alcohol is a strong predictor of suicide.

Alarming as it is, between 60-80% of those who die by suicide are intoxicated at the time of their death, 18-66% who die by suicide have some alcohol in their blood, and 23% of suicides are committed by those with a diagnosis of alcohol dependence. Marijuana is the most commonly detected drug in those who committed suicide, and contributes to the risk. Because so many contemporary alcoholics and drug addictions use multiple drugs, the likelihood of suicidal behavior is increased over past suicide attempts.

The association of alcohol and drugs with suicidal thinking and behavior is both causal and conductive. The subjective state of hopelessness is key to the disposition to actual suicides. Alcohol and drugs are influential in providing a feeling of hopelessness by their toxic effects, by possible manipulating of neurotransmitters responsible for mood and judgment and by disruption of interpersonal relationships and social supports. The identification of alcohol and drug use and dependence is critical to the proper assessment of suicide.

According to studies, over fifty percent of all suicides are associated with alcohol and drug dependence, and at least 25% of alcoholics and drug addicts commit suicide. Over 70% of adolescent suicides may be complicated by drug and alcohol use and dependence. Because alcoholism and drug addiction are leading risk factors for suicidal behavior and suicide, any alcoholic or drug addict should be assessed for suicide, especially if actively using.

Individuals with alcohol and drug addiction and prior aggressive behavior are more likely to report suicidal thoughts or past suicide attempts. Those who committed serious violent acts (rape, murder, assault) were more than twice as likely to report multiple suicide attempts. Recent violence was associated with increased likelihood of suicide. Suicide is a violent act against oneself, so the likelihood of violent acts against another is probable.

Yet many look under the rock for other causes of depression and suicidal behaviors than drugs and alcohol, and don't believe intoxicating sedation by depressant drugs cause the suicidal behaviors. There are many problems with that way of thinking. Nothing happens to the depression until the addicting drugs and alcohol are discontinued. Treating a so-called "underlying depression" does not alter the depression caused by the drugs. The patients are no help as they deny, minimize, and rationalize their drug use. Mysteriously, they think the drugs and alcohol are helping them cope with the depression, even treating the depression.

The "self-medication" hypothesis states that someone uses drugs and alcohol as a medication to treat the underlying depression. The problem is the depression gets worse with using increasing amounts of the drugs and alcohol. The hypothesis is based on a psychoanalytic view propagated by Sigmund Freud, who himself used cocaine at some point in his career and experienced depression. His theories were not empirically based as you can see. He postulated that everyone has a neurosis, or unconscious conflict, and some used drugs and alcohol to treat the neurotic anxiety and depression. He was right about some things, such as the defense mechanism, largely unconscious, that hide the addictions, and actually conspire to make the individual believe the opposite of what is true; that depressing drugs help, not hurt depression.

An experiment done at Harvard Medical School years ago showed the paradoxical effects of alcohol on mood and suicidal thinking. At the beginning, alcoholic subjects were asked why they drank, and often responded, "Because I am anxious and depressed." Curiously, they did not look or sound anxious and depressed, and did not complain of suicidal thoughts. Then, the researchers gave them alcohol and observed their mood and thoughts. Over days, the alcoholics became anxious and depressed as they drank more alcohol, and further complained of suicidal thoughts.

After the alcohol was discontinued and the alcoholics were detoxified, their mood normalized and found themselves no longer suicidal. The differences are: the intoxicating, depressant effects of alcohol, and how alcohol worsens, not improves, anxiety and depression. This scenario is played out thousands of times, daily, and continuously, and is the rule. It is not uncommon for alcoholics and drug addicts to think their drug treats depression. Even when suicidal.

Another story I like to tell illustrates the crazy addictive behavior that takes place. An alcoholic/addict sits outside a door. They hear a knock, and open the door. Someone with a bat hits them on the head. After they drop to floor, they get up and sit back in the chair. Another knock, and they open the door to get hit again. Another knock, and they open the door to get hit again. Another knock, and they open the door to get hit again. Another knock, and they open the door to get hit again. Another knock, and they open the door to get hit again. Another knock, and they open the door to get hit again. Another knock, and they open the door to get hit again. Another knock, and they open the door to get hit again. Another knock, and they open the door to get hit again. Another knock, and they open the door to get hit again. Another knock, and they open the door to get hit again. Another knock, and they open the door to get hit again. Another knock, and they open the door to get hit again.

One day the knocking stops. Guess what the addict does? Bet you can't. Instead of sitting peacefully, and reflecting, the alcoholic/addict opens the door and goes looking for the person with the bat. That is addiction in a nutshell. Not many understand those dynamics. Why would they? Very illogical. The addict obviously does not. Doctors do not. A mixture doomed to failure, destruction, and death.

Neither doctors nor therapists or really very many know or understand the relationship between drugs and mood. Combined with the twisted, self-destructive thinking, not much is accomplished to help the depressed alcoholic/drug addict if their addiction is not dealt with. The short answer is to confront the addict and discontinue the drug use before suicide occurs. Giving in to the distorted, delusional thinking induced by drugs prolongs the agony and risk for death.

For me, trying to diagnose drug and alcohol disorders in psychiatric populations is like Indiana Jones trying to avoid overwhelming odds from evil attacks, only I am not always as gifted, resilient, or lucky. I was more like Don Quixote chasing windmills, with only an individual effect, far short of changing the larger practices. I also carried the message, and truth was more the sword. As in politics, truth was not what people wanted, and prejudice and discrimination ruled. I needed dynamite to crack the distorted personal feelings and attitudes towards drug addiction and drug effects in treatment providers. Though I did make slow but sure progress in some settings, I was always swimming against the current, long distances between finding land, and taking in too much water. Fortunately, I survived when I had support from the top. Without such support, I frequently drowned.

Not sure how much politics help in addiction because of stigma and prejudice. It's notably hard to find much political support for dirt bags and moral lepers. Being short personally on politics to begin with didn't help my cause. Moreover, being relatively uncompromising in my views and opinions on addiction didn't help me to persuade institutions or the public. Patient lives were always more important to me than having a pleasing position that satisfied everyone's moral indignation. So I was willing to fight and lose, and fight again. I lost jobs because of my outspoken positions on addictions. But my determined approach did help my patients and publications.

I set up dual diagnosis programs on the psychiatric unit at UIC, which was like working in a hornet's nest. I upset a lot of people who are probably still mad today. I began working at a large psychiatric hospital where addiction was the elephant in the living room. Clinicians walked around it despite it being the predominant cause of psychiatric symptoms and admissions.

Personally, I could not bend or compromise the need for abstinence due to the loss of control over use of drugs and alcohol. I had to be rigid about abstinence. I had a hard time convincing that people do not drink or use drugs compulsively because of deep-rooted psychological problems or to escape, and they only become more trapped with the mounting adverse consequences from their addictive use.

Nurses told patients to complain about me because I tried to help them get off opioids. They accused me of not treating pain, yet they didn't know or understand much about opioid drugs in the first place. The nurses and patients were furious because I called them addicts. Not true! If anything, I said they were addicted or had an addiction. Though I would stop short of that diagnosis, just recommending they come off opioid medications to improve mood and decrease pain. As I said before, which many do not realize, is that opioid drugs actually increase pain through opioid induced hyperalgesia.

Seriously, I was called in to patient rights because a patient on high doses of Dilaudid complained about me. The patient was completely addicted to the narcotic, very depressed and suicidal, not working, early middle age. She was clueless about how narcotics incapacitated her. Upset because she thought I labeled her an addict, although I just focused on how opioids were causing her severe depression. Yet she kept using narcotics because she was addicted, not because the drugs were helping her. It's not like I am making things up, opioids are highly addicting even if prescribed for pain. Even by law, they're labeled a controlled substance because of their addicting properties.

315

Despite over 50% of patients admitted to psychiatric inpatient hospitals having drug and alcohol addiction, it was still something the clinician did not diagnose or treat. The psychiatrist just gave medications to treat depression and anxiety even though the actual treatment was to stop the addicting opioids, stimulants, tranquilizers, and alcohol. I noticed that many of the patients who complained about depression and psychosis had urine drug screens positive for marijuana, opioids, stimulants, benzodiazepines. I would say marijuana was the most common positive finding.

Marijuana, particularly the so-called "medical marijuana" version, is very potent these days, much stronger than years back. Marijuana has always been implicated in causing hallucinations and delusions, but much more with the high THC concentrations in medical marijuana. THC is tetrathydocarbinnol, the active ingredient that produces the effects that people seek. Today's marijuana contains 50% THC concentrations whereas it had less than 10% THC in the past. So, you can see why so many are excited about medical marijuana, a much bigger bang, with much more toxicity.

A hallucination is a false perception such as seeing objects, or people or pictures that don't exist in reality but do in the minds of the perceiving. A delusion is a fixed false belief that is incorrigible, idiosyncratic, and does not correspond to reality but may have a kernel of truth that germinated the delusion. Many of the hallucinations and delusions caused by marijuana vanished once the marijuana clears the brain because they are induced by the drug, and not mental illness.

In my personal and professional knowledge and experience, I have observed consistently paranoid thinking or delusions in marijuana users. Paranoia is fearful, apprehensive, threatening, persecutory thoughts, that someone or something is or will harm you. A feeling of impending doom and anxiety. Some people get it when they drink too much coffee (caffeine), and many experience paranoia from marijuana and other drugs such as stimulants.

Paranoia may also be a symptom of a mental illness such as schizophrenia or bipolar disorder. These mental illnesses commonly have paranoid delusions as part of their symptoms. The paranoid delusions are often persecutory, that someone is being harmed, victimized, harassed, and persecuted for no reason at all. Sometimes the delusions may take the form of grandiose beliefs, not corresponding to reality. Grandiose delusions are omnipotent, powerful, great thoughts, and beliefs of having super or special powers. Grandiose thinking arises from mental illness and drugs, often marijuana, stimulants, and other hallucinogenic drugs.

When I drank as I did, often and heavily, I had hangovers, god-awful feelings. I slept as long as I could, felt groggy, shaky, anxious, agitated, gloomy, clumsy, and my whole life was filled with dark, rainy days. I had little energy, motivation, or desire to complete tasks, could only accomplish the most basic mental and physical activities. I was just waiting until I could get the next drink, to be drunk. I either tried to wait because I could not get anything done drunk, but also because I was a total waste. I could not maintain drunkeness too long before I blacked and passed out. I did feel sick and that uncontrollable drive to get to the next drink.

For sure, I was depressed. I had the signs and symptoms of a depressive episode as defined in the Diagnostic and Statistical 5 (DSM-5), the Psychiatric bible for diagnosis. I had a depressed mood most of the day, nearly every day, and I drank nearly every day. I felt sad, empty, hopeless, and irritable. I had little pleasure or interests, weight gain, hypersomnia as I did not want to wake up to face myself or the day. I was constantly restless, fatigued, listless, no energy. I felt worthless, guilty, and you guessed it, "Lower than a batch of wet whale shit!" I couldn't think or concentrate, had feelings of wanting to die, and suicide attempts. These signs and symptoms of depression caused great stress and impairment in my social, school, work life, and other areas of my life. However, this depressive episode was attributable to the physiological effects of alcohol, and later drugs.

During one terrifying suicide attempt I was on a date with a nurse I had met on a medical service during my internship. I recall getting totally loaded, and driving her back at high speeds in a blackout, and then back to my apartment. I felt so depressed and intoxicated, I took a knife and tried to sever my left radial artery at the wrist. I learned it is not easy to actually commit suicide that way, and very painful. I can't remember who I called but someone came to my apartment and took me to the University of Michigan Hospital. I woke up the next morning on the orthopedic surgery service to a team of doctors headed by my Chairman. He said I had a disease like a broken leg, and needed treatment. He was a wonderful man.

The next near death incident was the time when I woke up on my sofa, which was on fire. When I was so intoxicated I merely threw the sofa out from my second story patio to the ground below, and went back to sleep. I woke up hours later to smoldering furniture. I was too drunk to even call the fire department. I really didn't care what happened to me, or anyone else, I guess. But I had enough sense to get rid of the fire, though not enough to care how. The next day I proceeded as though it was just another day, with not much worry about my previous escape from a fiery death.

Once I got onto drugs, I escalated my march towards near death with narcotics and sedatives. I had a terrible sleeping problem, and of course an addiction that required daily use of potent sedatives and narcotics. I was swallowing bottles of codeine (with Tylenol) that stimulated me, actually. So I had to come down with sedatives, Chloral Hydrate and Placidyl. These were potent enough to take down an elephant, I think!

Anyway, I liked to mix these drugs with alcohol to get a drunken, numb feeling. I had lost the intoxicating effects from alcohol alone. I was at the time a resident at the University of Chicago, and lived close to the hospital. One night I took a usual large amount of codeine, chloral hydrate, and Placidyl but had passed out close to my front door to the hallway. I had somehow left the door open, don't ask me how. I think God did it.

The next thing I knew I was wrapped in a straight jacket in the emergency room at the hospital where I was a resident, fighting with the staff trying to restrain me. I had woken up after my neighbors found me unconscious and unarousable on the floor after inviting themselves in through the open door. After the ER incident I woke up on the Psychiatric Floor of the hospital; a prelude to my Hopkins episode. I don't remember the diagnoses given to me. I do remember having God-awful anxiety and humiliation though. I could not seem to kill myself either intentionally or unintentionally. Which is a good thing, as it turned out. Though addicts deserve to die, don't they?

I remained anxious and depressed, taking drugs,

drinking, and an accident waiting to happen. My anxiety was paralyzing. I had tightness in my stomach, a terrific headache, and feelings of impending doom. Who wouldn't feel anxious if their behavior was unpredictable, dangerous, and lethal? I was out of control, on a roller coaster, with undulating sensations and a terrifying reality. I was restless, always on edge, fatigued, irritable, tense, needing drugs to sleep. These feelings pervaded my life, disturbed and impaired my social, work, and life in general. Life continued to be a "shit sandwich" and I struggled for another bite.

Not to mention, my poor judgment from my addictions. I had found my way yet to another residency in medicine. I was called to the emergency room one night or early in the morning more likely, to see an alcoholic patient I had previously treated on my inpatient medical service for alcoholic gastritis and near death from gastric bleeding. I looked down at him with blood all over him, and asked if he had been drinking. When he said yes, I immediately turned on my heels, and left the room. I called my supervising resident to take care of this patient and went to back to bed. I don't really remember what my resident said to me in the morning, but probably not, "Good job."

I had come to hate myself so deeply because of my drinking and drugging. I took my self-rage out on this patient. He symbolized my inability to take care of myself, to stop drinking, and harming myself. I was as furious with him as I was with myself. I loathed my basic being, and wanted to kill myself and others like me.

I will have to admit that most of my drug use up to this point was self-prescribed. I merely took out a prescription pad and wrote for my poisons. I did not have to make up excuses or illnesses to trick or coax doctors to prescribe my lethal drugs, though that would not be hard to do. I just reached into the candy jar and took whatever I wanted. I let my addiction do the thinking. And I kept doing the same things, and guess what, getting the same results, doom and destruction. Is not that insanity?

You have to understand how my personal experiences affect my professional life. I have suffered from many of the clinical problems my patients present to me with. I have had deep depression with feelings of helplessness and hopelessness, anxiety with apprehension and impending doom, and near delusional denial of my addictions and powerlessness over drugs. Having experienced drug induced near-death, and the harrowing battles and defeat from my addictions, I had many psychiatric symptoms and psychiatric consequences from my addictions.

I know first-hand what my patients are experiencing, and the risks and peril they face. I know how close to death they are from their drug use. They often don't. Through their denial, or disregard to the dangers with a cavalier, reckless defiance. Appearing to look over the abyss with a readiness to jump. The insanity of the addiction compels the addict to their unintended destiny.

I am often terrified and feel helpless when I hear and see what patients are doing to themselves with alcohol and drugs. I cannot convince them otherwise. Compounding my agony is their defensive, deluded response to my concern. They will say, "Alcohol helps me with my stress, I need Adderall to get through day, marijuana helps me cope, and the narcotics helps my pain." I hear these explanations while they are hospitalized for depression, anxiety, psychosis, suicidal behaviors. I try not to argue, but they often will cut me off as I try to give them a medical explanation. It's as if I am talking to the blind, deaf, and dumb.

I don't usually tell them I am a recovered alcoholic,

addict. I want them to accept my opinion based on medical knowledge and experience. They are seeking a physician's care, not a recovered addict. Besides, I can deliver my message medically. But medical knowledge and opinions do not penetrate the denial from addiction I face; though the patient may remember my medical advice and act on it later.

I cannot hold them in the hospital or make them accept treatment. I can only intervene if they are imminently at risk to harm themselves, then I have a duty to protect them from self-harm. Often that means involuntarily admitting them to the hospital against their will. That action does not always mean they will accept their addictions but it does give them a temporary reprieve from killing themselves.

Believe it or not, many psychiatric inpatient programs do not offer treatment for the addictive use of alcohol and drugs that drives the suicidal behavior. Rather sometimes providing detoxification, sometimes not, and the patient is left to suffer from untreated drug withdrawal, with its medical risks of seizures, delirium, and psychiatric risks of God awful anxiety, agitation, and suicidal depression and agony. The patient is left to suffer medically and psychiatrically. The hospital staff get paid for treating the "psychiatric symptoms," and addiction is not something psychiatric staff see themselves as needing to treat, even from the addictive use of drugs and alcohol.

Even worse, the patient is told that they have deep-rooted psychological problems, and psychiatric diagnosis such as underlying depression, anxiety, psychosis, are made. Liberal medications are usually given, often more addicting medications that not only further addictions and incapacitation, but also do not work to solve the source of the psychiatric impairment and life-threatening consequences from the addiction. Not only do these psychiatric treatment providers get away with these dangerous practices, but the third party providers or insurance companies do not pay for addiction treatment in inpatient psychiatric settings. Or even in addiction settings. While an inpatient psychiatric hospital stay may temporarily restrain someone from killing themselves, it does not alter course of their addiction or psychiatric consequences, and eventual death.

So a patient comes in suicidal and leaves suicidal, just not intoxicated yet. Not hard to understand why so many people die from drugs and alcohol. Not much useful treatment. Even when someone is identified or identifies themselves as a drug addict or alcoholic, there is minimal treatment available. Third party payers or insurance companies cover the costs for a few days of detoxification, maybe, and not much for residential treatment afterwards. There is more reimbursement available for mental health treatment, which is not generous either. The prognosis for addicts is generally good if treated, as they do not have serious, persisting mental illnesses from other causes whose prognosis is less promising.

I have published studies that show good outcomes for alcoholics and drug addicts. Abstinence rates at one year of 70-80% can be achieved with attendance at Alcoholics or Narcotics Anonymous. Further, if someone has attended regular meetings of AA for one year, they have an 80% chance of staying sober another year. And if abstinent in AA for five years, they have a 90% chance of staying sober another year. Long-term sobriety is common, and recovery in AA has many benefits besides just not drinking or drugging.

The 12 Steps are a plan for living, and therapy for personality, depression, and anxiety. Depression and anxiety are not only caused by direct effects of drugs and alcohol, but by how we live, conflicts in daily life, conscience, underlying urge or craving for alcohol and drugs, broken relationships, resentments. AA's 12 Steps help with living and mental conflicts that interfere with successful interpersonal relationships.

Although resentments are our number one offender and are a killer for addicts, they can be successfully dealt with on a personal basis in the 12 Steps, particularly, 4 through 10. Because addicts/alcoholics are always a risk for relapse to drugs and alcohol, maintaining an emotional balance, reducing conflict, anxiety and depression are vital to sustained recovery. Alcoholism and addictive disease is a spiritual, mental, physical malady. Maintaining spiritual fitness is essential to good living and abstinence through Steps 10 and 11. Maintaining mental balance is key to good relationships and abstinence. Of course, a good physical condition is necessary to health and prosperity.

A typical day in psychiatric hospital practice for me as a psychiatrist started with evaluating and filling out papers for involuntary hospitalization. I evaluated for the risk of harm to self and/or others, most often, suicidal statements or attempts. Obviously not completed suicide. Frequently the individual denies making such statements or minimizes the attempt, "I am just seeking attention" or "They didn't understand what I meant." Involuntary hospitalization is like incarceration, though not for punitive reasons, but to protect individual from harm to self or others. Being physically incarcerated against their will is by definition involuntary. Some decide it is a good idea, others fight it, but most comply to some extent either to get out or get help.

Many new admissions have alcohol and drug problems, some have additional psychiatric problems. Over half of those with a diagnosis of Schizophrenia use marijuana, often times along with alcohol or other drugs. Those diagnosed with Bipolar Disorder also have similar high rates of comorbid drug use. But I can't always tell for sure if they are having symptoms from alcohol and drugs, simply Bipolar illness, or both. Even if both, their symptoms will improve as they detoxify from the alcohol and drugs. Then, I can sometimes tell the difference because their depression, anxiety, or psychosis will improve within a few days if they are due to drugs and alcohol. The symptoms for Schizophrenia and Bipolar Disorder will persist longer, and often not resolve completely even with treatments. But the symptoms will improve as they detoxify from drugs and alcohol.

Marijuana commonly causes violent behaviors, psychosis, anxiety, depression, in those with and without mental illnesses. Marijuana is actually classified as a hallucinogen, and today's high potency marijuana is even more likely to produce transient symptoms of mental illness in otherwise normal individuals. Making mood, hallucinations and delusions worse in those with Schizophrenia, Bipolar Disorder, depression, or anxiety disorders.

Adderall is dextroamphetamines and causes psychosis, delusions, hallucinations, and paranoia. Adderall is "speed," and "speed kills." So does Adderall. It is a highly dangerous and addicting drug. It's prescribed for Attention Deficit Disorder. But it turns out to be another drug like methamphetamines, or "ice," chemically very similar. Yet one is legal, and the other not. Why? Doctors and drug companies. Big Pharma brainwash already dull doctors about addicting drugs. Selling Adderall to the public is big business and profits, even if it doesn't work or is debilitating and lethal. Profits, not lives, matter. Doctors like it because they can improve their patient satisfaction scores and make money as well. Every visit makes money, and it takes less than five minutes to write and hand a prescription to a demanding addict. While, to deny writing a prescription attracts negative responses, and low satisfaction scores.

The federal government has decided that patients always know what's best for them. Therefore, Medicare and Medicaid base reimbursement on patient satisfaction. And patient satisfaction accounts for 25% of the total ratings used for reimbursement. If patient satisfaction scores are low, reimbursement may be low or denied. The government, in its limited understanding of medical care and intrusive meddling in doctor-patient relationships, fosters drug addiction to new levels; paving the way to patient death and destruction.

It's beyond me that a bureaucrat, miles away from the doctor and patient can prescribe and monitor medical care. Will they understand that low satisfaction scores and negative reviews of medical care by a drug addict is misleading and an unhealthy response to an appropriate refusal to prescribe dangerous and disabling medications? Just imagine the angry response and low scores from a rejected addict. I know first hand from satisfaction scores I get, when I try to explain to someone addicted that the medications they are taking are harmful and not effective. I often get a very personal response.

Does the government care? It doesn't. It just follows rules governing entitlements and medical necessity by law, not evidence based medicine. It has disability programs that dissatisfied patients can apply for and obtain disability. Even though their disability is caused by an ineffective and addicting medication, and even though their disability will cease with discontinuation of the medications, these patients often are awarded money indefinitely.

Pharma likes selling addicting drugs because addiction is perfect compliance, and drug addicts will buy their drugs even though they are being harmed by them. Pharma could care less about disabling people or even killing them for that matter. Their sole objective is profit and greed. You'd think deaths are bad for business for drug companies, since they are lost customers. But there are far more live addicts than dead addicts, though not small in numbers. Doctors will yield even if they understand the harmful medications because they too make a profit, and addicts deserve bad outcomes, even death, because addicts cause their own problems. After all, addicts do not have a disease, they have a moral problem. Worse yet, doctors don't know better, they are not educated or trained enough in addictions or addicting medications.

So you say this is contemporary medical care? I say yes. I know it from both ends. Is it frightening? Very, as seen by someone who knows you can suffer and die from this kind of care. What can we do? Get honest, focus on good patient care, include addiction in medical care, and don't let profits and government kill people. Learn about addiction and mental illness and their true relationship. And force medical schools and residencies to train doctors about addictions, which they don't do now.

I was removed from a Medical Consultation Service because social workers and physicians, who wanted to prescribe opioids, complained about me. I was very popular with other Hospitalist Physicians treating the patients. Consultation requests increased dramatically for me to help treat drug and alcohol addictions, detoxification, and referral for treatment. Complaints stemmed more from clinicians who did not like my emphasis on addiction. Addiction was still a bad word, stigma high, and the patient's fault.

And prejudice won out.

Physicians take little responsibility for prescribing addicting medications or diagnosing alcohol and other drug problems. They blame these problems on the patients, even though the patients could not control their use. It's like knowingly prescribing penicillin to someone who is allergic, and blaming them for the allergy. Only works in addictions where the patient is at fault, and the physician is excused. Prejudice against the patient for having addictive diseases.

Body language can tell a lot. I already felt different in groups. I felt that the spotlight was on me because I wanted to diagnose and treat addicted patients. I felt isolated and alone. People may agree with me but would not openly support me. I made little progress on my own. I could make progress if I had other support. Otherwise, I would not die on the vine. Nonetheless, I continued to make new fronts to improve care in addictions.

Don't you know it's hard to fight and not even know why
Don't you know it's hard to try and keep on losing

—"Don't You Know" Clockwork Orange

20

MEDICAL DISEASES:
ADDICTION, DISABILITY, DEATH

"Doctors are the same as lawyers, the sole difference being that lawyers only rob you, but doctors rob you, and kill you too..." —Anton Chekhov

I self-prescribed and administered 20 to 40 Darvon (propoxyphene) 100mg pills per day. I lost 50 lbs. or more. I subsisted on yogurt and sweetbread. I was so constipated that I had to de-impact myself with gloves. I acted strangely towards others but no one ever took a urine drug screen to detect drugs. I also combined the narcotics with valium, 40-60 mg a day, and Placidyl, a potent sedative. I was pretty bombed on this cocktail. I didn't take it for pain, but for my cunning, baffling, powerful, and mysterious drug addictions. It led to my near fatal overdose. Now that I don't prescribe these drugs for myself, I apply my first-hand knowledge to others who suffer from addiction to medications from whatever cause. Because I am a physician, I often work in doctor patient populations. Unfortunately, in today's medical practice, doctors are quite willing to support and sustain drug addictions.

In medical work with patients, I practice Step 12, "Having had a spiritual awakening of the result of these steps, we tried to carry this message to alcoholics (drug addicts), and to practice these principles in all affairs." I certainly identified with patients addicted to narcotic medications, and was scared to death what would happen to them because of what happened to me. I had reached death, only to escape. I had to carry my message to patients addicted to narcotic medications and help them save their lives. Help them to avoid so many medical consequences, disability, and other unnecessary, harmful medical treatments. I carried a message of truth, though certainly not popular despite being life-saving. I was a target, not a prophet. The problem, not the solution.

You wouldn't believe how medical practice treats addiction and addicted patients. Drug and alcohol addiction is almost totally ignored in medical education and residency training. Making up a small fraction of their medical education, if any. Most doctors have no idea what drug addiction is, think obesity and cigarette smoking are life style choices, and addiction as a disease is foreign to them. These deaths are not medical matters and do not matter to doctors. And so the patient is blamed. They do it to themselves. But guess what? Doctors do not even ask about these causes of death, don't mention them to their patients, don't even advise them to avoid them.

Cigarette smoking, which is a nicotine addiction, kills 400,000 people a year, obesity kills 500,000 per year, alcohol kills 100,000 per year, and drug addiction 60,000 per year. Almost a million deaths a year are attributable to addictive diseases: drugs, alcohol, and food addictions, out of a total of 2,500,000 deaths per year. Some form of addiction kills upwards towards half of our population, and medically, you would think doctors would be fired up and eager to treat and prevent deaths due to addiction. That's a Hippocratic Oath they took to first, "Relieve suffering and do no harm."

Sadly, that is far from the truth and medical practice.

I was harassed for being insensitive to pain. I would evaluate patients having subjective complaints of extreme pain, 10 out of 10, where 10 is the worst pain they have experienced. Interestingly, they did not show much pain behavior such as moving around, avoiding reproducing pain, mostly just demanding narcotic pain medications. Claiming nothing else worked than Vicodin, or OxyContin, or Morphine. Their descriptions of their pain was often graphic, yet inconsequential, and not a sufficient explanation for pain. "I have degenerated discs in my back." Who doesn't, I ask? Most of the U.S. population above the age of 30 has degenerative joint disease. Or they are repeating what their doctor may have told them? Many have not actually had their pain evaluated with MRI or CT scans, and if they did, the results were often negative or mild and minimal abnormalities.

Importantly, why would a patient or doctor want to continue a treatment that did not relieve pain as a 10/10, where 10 is the worst pain, when it is not ultimately working as pain relief? Wouldn't you think to stop prescribing narcotic medications and try something else? I served as an expert witness in a large-scale lawsuit against Purdue-Pharma pharmaceutical company for false claims regarding the narcotic medication, OxyContin (oxycodone). Purdue-Pharma was flooding the market with the dangerous and highly addicting drug, and consequent disability and death.

While I was reviewing medical records of patients who were prescribed large doses of OxyContin and complaining of 10/10 pain, I asked myself, why does the doctor continue to prescribe and the patient take the drug? It is not because OxyContin relieved pain, rather it is because it is addicting-compulsive use, despite adverse consequences.

As you now know, narcotic medications actually paradoxically increase pain over time (opioid-induced hyperalgesia), and there is no evidence they are effective in long-term management of chronic pain. *Why would anyone want to continue a treatment that made the pain worse?* Someone addicted. Addicted is a painful state, and made worse by narcotic medications. Unfortunately, doctors don't understand either, opioid drugs or addiction. Yet they are allowed to prescribe addicting medications with the rationalization of treating pain, as if pain is a bad thing itself.

Pain is protective. It warns us that there is a problem and motivates us to solve the problem. Without pain we could not survive. Treatment with narcotic medications is not to solve the underlying pain problem and actually makes us not care about the pain. Opioids dull the perception of pain and do not do anything about the underlying pain source. Thus, we don't care about increasing pain from opioids, pain that is much greater than the original pain, and creates pain everywhere in the entire body, and not just at the source.

The only way to understand why the patient complains of pain while on narcotics, is to understand addiction and the pharmacology or how the drug works. Since physicians receive little education and training in either, they don't know why their prescribing is not working. And guess what? They blame it on the patient.

Physicians rarely take responsibility for their prescribing these drugs and their disabling, painful, and lethal consequences. The patient wanted the medications, so I gave it to them. If physicians took responsibility for prescribing addicting and painful medications, they not only would stop prescribing the medications and blaming the patient, they would relieve pain and suffering. Something they seem more intent on creating than solving. If physicians practiced evidence-based medicine in regards to opioid medications, we would not have nearly the problems we're currently suffering from. The evidence is out there, just ignored; not something physicians and medical schools are interested in. The patient can solve their problem since it's their fault. And the physician will give them the opportunity.

When I worked on an addiction detoxification unit and was responsible for detoxifying patients from alcohol and other drugs, I was faced with the challenge of what to do for patients who also were prescribed narcotic medications by doctors for "pain." Because the narcotic medications are addicting, I naturally reasoned the patients needed to discontinue them. I had never seen in my doctor days where addicting narcotic medications taken compulsively and regularly ever helped anyone, even for pain. Besides, despite being on heavy doses of narcotics, they still had significant pain. And often I could not find or diagnose significant causes or sources of pain.

So, I was faced with patients taking addicting, depressing, and disabling medications requesting detoxification from other addicting drugs and alcohol. And narcotic medications work just like heroin, act at the same receptors, make people feel the same way, and produce irrational addictive, compulsive drug use. I decided to discontinue the narcotic medications as I would heroin or any other addicting drugs.

My staff nearly revolted. They said, "How can you discontinue these pain medications in patients taking them for pain and prescribed by doctors?" I said to myself and them, that addicts always have rationalizations or excuses for their drug use, such as: "I drink alcohol because I am depressed and anxious," "I need Xanax because I have anxiety," or "I need Adderall because I can't concentrate." When I examine them, their anxiety is through the roof and concentration is way off. Then why do they still want these drugs if they are not improving their symptoms? Answer again, is addiction.

So I told my staff that I would discontinue narcotic medications because their pain was very high, as continuing the medications would not solve their pain problem anyway. And discontinuing the medications may solve their pain problems. But neither the staff nor the patients were sold on the idea. It didn't help that the patients complained bloody murder at having to give up all their addicting drugs. Addicts fight that strategy even if it means not getting better, being in less pain, not depressed, sleeping better, improved sex life, increased appetite.

I continued to take patients complaining of pain off narcotics, and over time my staff found out that their pain complaints were down. Inexplicably, they had less pain without narcotics. So when the patients complained about being taken off narcotics, even if they looked and acted better, the staff knew and understood they were dealing with addiction, not pain behaviors. Eventually, I worked with a resident who became interested in the pain problem, and was struck with how the pain scales dropped.

The Joint Commission of Hospital Accreditation required hospitals to ask the patient for their level of pain, just subjectively. They required we use a 10 point scale, from 0 for no pain to 10 being the worst pain ever. I knew instinctively that this was a bad thing and would lead to more narcotic addiction, as it did eventually. But in our patients, the pain scores went down as we detoxified patients from the narcotic medications. Significantly lower pain scores meant the patients were in less pain after stopping the narcotic medications.

When I published these results, I had to review the medical literature for opioid medications. I found others had published findings that opioid medications actually caused pain when taken for a period of time, and called it "opioid induced hyperalgesia." Opioid is the term for narcotic pain medications and hyperalgesia means increased pain. Hyper meaning increased and algesia is pain. These results were published in national, prestigious medical journals as early as 2001. You would think doctors would read and care about these results. But sadly, no.

Studies show that total annual cost burden for a patient with an opioid abuse or dependence diagnosis was significantly higher than that for a patient with no such diagnosis, due to high rates of comorbidities, and utilization of medical services. The total annual charges associated with an individual who was diagnosed with opioid abuse or dependence were 56% higher than the average annual per-patient charge based on patients' charges. In 2015, the average per patient charge across all diagnoses and claims was $11,404. Comparatively, the per patient average total charge for patients identified with opioid diagnosis in the same year was $63,356.

Patients in hospitals receive narcotic medications whether they need them or not. It is standard practice to start with Dilaudid or Vicodin on admission, whether the patient wants it or not. Some patients seek it out and even pursue fraudulent medical and psychiatric care to get narcotics. It seems doctors and hospitals make money off addicts as they increase their pain by prescribing opioid medications. Doctors and hospitals figure out that they make money from knowingly admitting and treating addicts for the consequences of their addictions. And they don't even have to identify and treat the addictions. What is the incentive beyond good medical care to discontinue prescribing opioid medications?

In fact, there is great incentive to increase prescribing opioid drugs to escalate medical utilization and costs from the opioid medications, and certainly to continue providing narcotic medications to supplement the bottom line. All in the name of pain, even if not prescribing decreases pain. Why is it so hard to get doctors and hospitals to do the right thing? The answer is: money driven by addiction and ignorance.

Also, because the medications cause pain instead of reducing pain, physicians (particularly pain specialists), perform expensive procedures such as injections that have no medical value against opioid induced hyperalgesia. These procedures carry their own risks such as spinal infections, paralysis, increased pain. These procedures are on top of the money these doctors make for prescribing the narcotics in the first place, another money maker. Pain doctors charge $1000 to $2000 per injections that take 10 minutes, and does no good as the pain problem is narcotics. Injections don't work for opioid addiction.

Figure it out. A doctor charges $100 per a 10 minute visit to prescribe Vicodin or OxyContin, and sees 6 people per hour, 8 hours a day. That is $900 per hour or $4,800 per day, or $24,000 per 5-day week, and $1,152,000 for a 48-week year. No wonder doctors and hospitals prescribe narcotics. What happened to medical ethics? The same thing that happened to pharmaceutical industry aka Big Pharma: namely greed, and more greed. Prescribing opioid medications is a nifty way to make tons of money at the patient's expense and well-being. Not to mention the costs to our in-surance rates, Medicare, and Medicaid.

Hydrocodone, a narcotic medication, is the most commonly prescribed medication of any kind, greater than insulin, even antibiotics. And it has been for many years. Hydrocodone is a highly addicting medication, similar to heroin, so it is no small wonder that it is greatly sought after. Remember addiction is a powerful, instinctive drive; that we seek compulsively addicting drugs to the extent of loss of liberty, life, and happiness. In fact, as many as 16,000 people die a year from opioid medications and 12,000 die a year from heroin. That's 28,000 deaths from opioid drugs. Are they really worth it? When they don't have benefit, don't decrease pain, rather increase pain and cause disability and death?

Other reasons that hydrocodone is so commonly prescribed is pain is very common, and is a major reason people seek medical care. I know I have sought medical care for pain on occasions. Often the type of pain is chronic. Sources of pain are muscle, skeletal, headaches commonly. A set up for developing an addiction to opioid medication. Most people will develop an addiction to opioid medications if taken for weeks or months, if pain is chronic, and the risk for onset of addiction is high. Accordingly, addiction to opioid medications is the second most common drug addiction next to marijuana in the U.S. People of all ages become addicted. But the most common reason for becoming addicted is seeking medical care, for common sources of incurable pain. Yet opioids bring no comfort, rather discomfort.

I performed peer reviews on patients who were addicted to narcotic medications prescribed by physicians. Also, I reviewed dangerous and fraudulent prescribing of medications that were not medically necessary. Patients were on large doses of Vicodin (hydrocodone), Percocet (oxycodone), Duragesic (fentanyl). Because of addiction to the narcotics, the patients wanted to remain on the drugs. Because the doctors knew very little about these medications, they either didn't know much about what the patients were experiencing or didn't care. Also, doctors and hospitals profited. All they focused on was the patient's complaint of pain, and their demands to get more drugs. Physicans were intimidated or entrepreneurs. They also didn't know about the addictions that drove the patients' demands and use. They were clueless that the opioids caused pain. Because of complaints from physicians and companies, I was terminated from further reviews. Unfortunately, it looked like careless and dangerous patient driven, and not scientifically based physicians controlling the prescribing.

Patient satisfaction and addiction drive this type of care despite painful and dangerous outcomes. The US government requires patient satisfaction as a part of medicare reimbursement. If addicted patients complain (and they do), providers may not receive payments. Also, because providers depend on high volumes of patients to cover high overhead, they don't want to discourage patient utilization. Addictive use of drugs is perfect compliance because of its compulsive use, and can be billed for prescribing opioids.

I also do Independent Medical Evaluations for disability and medical necessity for patient care. It is not unusual to review cases where continuous prescribing of narcotic medications goes on for years. The claimants continue to receive large doses of multiple opioid medications for complaints of pain, which is really disguised addiction. The so-called pain specialists merely dole out narcotics, appearing clueless that the medications are causing pain, disability, and poor functioning. Attorneys who file personal injury and workers compensation claims, have favorite doctors they can count on to make such disabling diagnoses and to prescribe debilitating narcotic medications.

Narcotics are disabling because they lead to loss of function, poor quality of life, disruption of interpersonal relationships, unemployment, depression, anxiety, and increase rather than decrease pain. Imagine the costs of unnecessary medical care for medications, doctor visits, surgeries and what that does to costs of health insurance and government health programs.

Patients also use marijuana that is not really a pain medication. Marijuana causes anxiety, depression, delusions, disability, and debilitation. There is scant evidence that it reduces pain. It's just another drug that people become addicted to and use pain as a political and personal front to obtain marijuana for addictive use. There is virtually no evidence that marijuana is an effective analgesic or that it reduces pain beyond intoxication. And intoxication is a painful state.

Patients become further debilitated from the combination of opioids and benzodiazepine medications. Both are scheduled as controlled substances and dangerous drugs, and cause lethal unintentional and intentional overdoses. Users become suicidal and depressed and will take opioids and benzodiazepine drugs to kill themselves. Or they will unintentionally suffer from an overdose death from respiratory depression and ceased breathing. Because opioid medications cause anxiety and depression, doctors do not stop prescribing medications. Rather they add fuel to the fire by prescribing so called anti-anxiety medications like Xanax (alprazolam) or Valiam (diazepam). These medications set up a painful dependence and withdrawal that causes severe anxiety and depression. Because Xanax has a short half-life, people on it wake up at night in withdrawal for their next fix.

A large study done on Medicare and Medicaid recipients on government Social Security disability payments, found significant opioid prescribing, between 6 and 13 prescriptions per year in over one million enrollees. The big question they asked was, why? Since there was scant evidence provided for prescribing this amount of medications over this period of time. The costs to tax payers and the public are staggering and unnecessary. Add this to the costs to the individual, which are reversible and unnecessary, except death. Since most of the disability is caused by the narcotic drug itself, discontinuing it would result in loss of disability or more normal function. Off narcotics, the individual could be employed, in less pain, have less depression and anxiety, have better relationships and quality of life. You ask, why not? In my experience, my answer is addiction of the individual and profit by doctors, and Big Pharma. But don't forget the savings to the government and us.

In my review of medical records, on occasion the drug screens are negative, indicating the patients are not taking the medication, and the physicians continues to prescribe the medications. The clinical notes look like copies from electronic medical records from month to month, week to week with no change in diagnosis or treatment. The market value is high to sell hydrocodone, and chronic users or those obtaining prescriptions may try to sell the drugs for profit. Why not, everyone else is. One pill may sell for $10 or more, so a typical prescription for 60 tablets would yield $600, a nice monthly sum, given how easy doctors prescribe these drugs. The amount still pales on comparison to the millions and billions doctors, hospitals, and drug companies make off prescriptions.

Now that Big Pharma, doctors, and hospitals have made billions by only exploiting the suffering and death of patients from selling and prescribing opioids; there's more to be made from addicting the public to marijuana. Big Pharma is salivating over the enormous profits from selling yet another addicting drug, already widely used. Doctors and hospitals already know how much medical care addicting drugs generate in profits from increased medical care.

Of course, the government, politicians, and bureaucrats spend sleepless nights trying to find bigger and better ways to go deeper in debt. Not only do I not want to pay for unnecessary medical care, disability, government debt, and greed from medical pharmaceutical industrial complex, I also don't want people to suffer and die from senselessly smoking weed and using narcotics. More debt, death, pain. The cycle continues with addiction as the driving engine of fatal outcomes.

Politics again. I was working on a consultation service in a major hospital in Grand Rapids. I actually was providing psychiatric and addiction consultative services. The demand for my services grew dramatically, as many of the hospitalists caring for patients were foreign and did not understand why patients should receive addicting opioid medications. They saw right through the drug seeking behaviors and their influence on the medical care. The hospitalists made me a very popular consultative doctor. I had large numbers of requests to diagnose and treat opioid addiction in addition to the usual patients with alcohol detoxification and referral for treatment.

Then out of the blue one day, I was called into my medical director's office and told my consultative services were no longer needed. I was very perplexed but frankly getting accustomed to being yanked abruptly over something related to addictions, especially if I was really helping patients and making a difference. This was just yet another occasion. He explained the chief of the medical staff called to say he did not want my services any longer, without an explanation.

Here I was, in the peak of my popularity at the hospital, helping doctors and patients, now unceremoniously forced out without regard to how much I was helping others. These decisions were certainly not based on patient benefit, rather prejudice and bias towards me personally. I later found out that one physician, well situated in the administrative hierarchy, was able to unilaterally persuade the chief medical officer to "can" me without due process or regarding to patient care. Without success, I was not able to confront this chief about it as he refused any such meeting with me. Only in addictions would such unprofessional treatment occur towards another professional, leaving the patient to suffer as usual.

This incident was not the last to happen to me. I was still working on a consult service at another hospital. With my reputation as being disruptive, I faced more consequences of trying to help doctors and patients with opioid addictions. I was removed from yet another consult service because of complaints about recommending patients come off narcotic medications. I was told, "All hell breaks loose when you recommend stopping narcotic medications, and it takes time to resume order." Not only did patients complain of me, but also social workers who made personal attacks on me such as, "He speaks so loud," "The family is upset the patient is not on narcotic medications," and "The patient is complaining of pain."

Everyone wants more drugs, dismissing any ideas that these were dangerous and disabling, and interfering with medical care that relieved pain and suffering. I was unceremoniously removed from that consultative service despite some popularity with nurses and other professionals. As always, moves to dismiss me were swift, without much review, and certainly not based on medical facts about opioid drugs. Facts didn't matter. Just get rid of someone in the way of opioid addiction, even if they know what they are talking about, even if they are helping patients.

Just to convince you the bias and prejudice aren't rare in the medical profession and is really systematic, I have another experience to share from medical school. I had been hired as a professor in a newly formed medical school to work in addictions of all things. I got a little too pushy I think, for a dean and a few others. I had been asked by the person who hired me, to develop a curriculum in addictions in a neuroscience course for the second year medical students. I also wanted to serve on the curriculum committee for the school of medicine. I asked the Dean of the Medical School to appoint me over the head of the Dean of the Committee, who did not want me on the committee. It didn't take the curriculum dean long to terminate my "at will" contract.

This time I was informed my contract was done and was escorted out of the medical school by a security officer for reasons not given to me. I recall everyone staring at me in the halls, in wonder of why I required such security. Someone took the extra effort to make me look bad, and certainly did a good job. To be honest, I was only too happy to leave such a crazy place. However, it was with regrets. The medical students did not get education in addiction. This particular dean in charge of medical student education made sure that didn't happen in grand style.

Yet, there is more to this story. The school eventually hired a new Dean of the Medical School. He happened to be very interested in addictions, having set up addiction programs previously. This is *the* Dean mind you. He wanted me to establish addiction education in the neuroscience course. I am a natural to do that as I am a neurologist, psychiatrist, and addiction psychiatrist, ready to develop education curriculum for medical students who otherwise would remain nave to knowledge and skill in addictive diseases. Well, guess what? The previous curriculum dean rose to the position of Dean of Faculty, and was once again, able to block again any appointment of me by him. Here I am again, held back from educating doctors in addictions; a continuing conspiracy to keep them ignorant and in the dark. The deans were good soldiers in supporting and carrying out this agenda.

Now you ask, why do we have so many problems with addicting medications and an opioid epidemic? One that involves such widespread death and destruction from opioid drugs? You have the answers from my experience. You have enough information to decide for yourself. If doctors are kept stupid about addicting drugs, and there are medications commonly prescribed by doctors, and pain is the most common reason patients seek medical care in primary care physicians' practices, an equation is satisfied. That equation I dreamt up, namely: availability plus vulnerability equal addiction. Undereducated doctors kept in the dark about narcotics, who already have the built in prejudice towards anyone who becomes addicted, are prime sources for the drugs themselves.

Vulnerability is really the susceptibility to become addicted. Most people have inherent susceptibility to become addicted in centers in the brain. Contrary to popular opinion, we have not yet found brain locations for morals. We have found areas in the brain that are responsible for reinforcement and compulsive, addictive use of drugs, the mesolimbic area. Drugs act on receptors and neurotransmitters to initiate and sustain addictive drug use. Also, it does seem that some who become addicted have genetic predispositions, therefore, genes that program for addictions. Thus, drug addiction is a brain disease with identifiable brain structures and locations. Yet how many doctors know about that, and how many medical schools teach it? Well, few and far between.

Most people see a doctor at some point, and many complain of pain. Doctors are readily accessible sources of addicting drugs. Add to that the public's interest in having addicting pain medications available, as they do addicting substances in general, and you have an avalanche of drugs available to virtually anyone. Pervasive to prescribing is the current entitlement in medical care, where pain is not permissible and narcotics are viewed as powerful pain medications. Even if not true. Add to that, the attitude that addiction is a personal choice, and under perfect control of the patient, then what's the worry? If they lose control over addicting drugs, it is a moral problem, unrelated to the pharmacological or inherent chemical addictive properties of narcotics. Morality is substituted for medical facts, and the patient is blamed for medical properties that the physician should be responsible for, namely high addiction potential, located in the patient's brain, not morals.

We are now in the midst of a predictable opioid epidemic. I anticipated and wrote about the coming problems a decade ago. I knew what was going to happen if anyone just looked at the facts, and medical history. Sure enough, it happened. But the real cause is not yet being talked about, namely doctor ignorance about the addicting drugs and people's moral view of addiction.

What's even more surprising is opioids are not particularly effective pain medications. When opioid medications are compared to other non-narcotic medications for effectiveness, opioid medications are the least effective in pain relief. Other medications often help the underlying source of pain by reducing inflammation. Whereas opioids do nothing to alter the pain, except increase it over time via opioid induced hyperalgesia.

I evaluated so many patients complaining of high levels of pain who were not open to alternatives treatments. To me, that's insanity, to do the same thing and expect different results. Any other treatments than addicting medications, the patient would gladly try a different treatment. But addicting drugs' power is to drive the patients to continue to use the medications compulsively, despite lack of reduced pain, and in fact more pain.

In opioid addicted patients, I often hear, "My Norco is the only the thing that helps the pain," yet their subjective level of pain is high, at the top. If pain relief were their goal, I would expect them to be open to stopping the narcotic and trying something else. I can explain that narcotic medications increase the risk for unintentional lethal overdose without seeing the patient flinch. And they ask for more Norco, acting as if there is no danger to more narcotic medications, and they are the only answer to pain.

If you think about it, the issue is not pain relief, rather drug seeking to satisfy the addictive drive to use more regardless of the pain. Addiction is only one of the reasons why narcotics are bad medications for chronic pain. Other reasons are opioid drugs alter the perception of pain subjectively to decrease or increase over time. In acute or short-term management, opioids can be effective in reducing pain, mostly by reducing the perception of pain. A typical reaction is, "I can feel the pain, but I don't care;" patient apathy towards the pain. An apathetic response is not always good because there may be disregard to protect from continuing injury or poor motivation to treat the underlying source of pain. I typically ask the patient if they have had a medical evaluation of the pain, particularly recent, and in view of their continuing high levels of pain complaints. "Oh no, I have not seen a doctor or not recently and have not tried anything but the Norco. It is the only thing that works for my pain."

Sometimes correction of the underlying pain is possible, whereas addiction to the narcotic interferes with good judgment to do something about the pain. In my personal case, I had almost crippling pain in my hip and back. I did not take narcotic medications because I wanted to avoid an even worse problem and reactivate my hopeless addiction, and not even lessen the pain. I eventually got hip replacement surgery. And I had a remarkable experience when I awoke from the surgery. The awful pain I had experienced for years was gone! Mind you, I had just had my bones sawed and nailed from the surgery, but I could tell the problem was taken care of. While I was doped up from the narcotics I was given during and immediately after surgery, I felt the arthritic, diseased bone was no longer there.

I was asked by the anesthetist just before the surgery if I wanted OxyContin during the procedure and I said, "Yes, if it keeps me from waking up." I do think narcotic medications are important and even necessary to administer acutely to facilitate surgeries but not indefinitely. I recall I did not take narcotics after discharge. I wanted to monitor my hip postoperatively, to protect it, and know if the surgery was successful. I was warned about developing blood clots in my legs that could go to my lungs to stop my breathing. I had to move around, keep active, exercise to prevent the clots from forming. Which is notably hard to do if I am sedated from a drug that makes me not care of the pain. In my instance, I wanted pain to be a motivation to protect my new hip from dislocation too. Without the pain warnings, I could damage my hip or fall while on intoxicating narcotics.

When I visited my surgeon for a follow up, I asked when I could drive, and they said when I no longer took narcotics. Since I wasn't taking narcotics, I could drive. In fact, two weeks after my second hip replacement, I drove to Chicago to testify as an expert witness in a trial, about four hours in the car. I was able to walk on the streets in downtown Chicago with a cane. Sitting in the witness stand was not easy, as I still had some pain from the surgery. However, I never could have accomplished this feat if I had been taking narcotic medications.

Another behavior that indicates addiction to narcotics is compulsiveness. The patient will take the narcotic like clockwork, routinely. So that the use of the drug is linked to properties of the drug and not the pain. Most narcotic medications have short half-lives, meaning their effects wear off within a few hours when withdrawal begins.

Withdrawal is an unpleasant feeling, which prompts more narcotic use to treat the withdrawal, and pain is a symptom of withdrawal. In other words, the narcotic use is linked to the drug, and not pain, and you can track it according to the pharmacologic or chemical properties. Complaints of pain from narcotic medications are general, not specific, vague, and do not often correspond to another cause other than the drug. If you follow the pain pattern, it will match the drug characteristics, and not any reasonable pattern of pain. You might say the pain relief from the drug wears off, but then you are saying the pain is constant, unremitting, unchanging, and not many types of pain fit that category. Most types of chronic pain vary with movement, position, and the underlying source of pain.

Another obvious clue to narcotic addiction is that the patient will complain vigorously of pain subjectively, but not show it objectively. Meaning they will say, "My pain is a 10 out of 10," yet they do not look in pain. They do not show pain behaviors. Someone with a 10 or worst possible pain, should be writhing in pain, unable to tolerate almost anything. Yet they can sit, walk, talk, smile, laugh, almost do anything, except go without the narcotic drug. The most pronounced behavior is drug seeking, wanting the drug, and more drug, and their subjective complaints dominate any objective evidence of pain. I like to say their lips move and say most anything to get the drug, reflecting the addictive drive for it.

If doctors only could understand and identify addictive behaviors, recognize the pharmacological and properties of narcotic medications, and evaluate pain behaviors, patients would ultimately get actual pain relief. I say I am a pain specialist because I recognize pain from addiction to narcotics. When I detoxify someone from narcotic medications, their pain improves quite dramatically, particularly if I treat the addictive drive to use the narcotic. If I don't treat the addiction, the patients may continue to complain of pain.

Although marijuana is the most commonly used addictive drug, next to alcohol, until recently its source has been illicit. Bought off the streets, illegally, limited the access and amount of marijuana available to users. With the onset of the ridiculous and unfounded so called, "medical marijuana" laws, the flood gates are open and just about everybody can get marijuana by just saying, "Ouch" or "I hurt." I can't really see where marijuana is medical, as no doctor treats the pain problem, rather a special marijuana doctor just signs a card and says goodbye. There is otherwise no doctor evaluation of the pain problem, no follow up by the doctor, no Federal Drug Administration (FDA) approval of marijuana as a medicine, no pharmacy to dispense it. Furthermore, there is no standard dosing, no informed consent for the toxic effects.

"Medical marijuana" is just smoking marijuana grown in someone's backyard. No FDA oversight for purity, effectiveness, or safety. Caregivers grow it, bundle it, and prepare it for smoking with no standards. What else can you think of that is sold "medically" to the public with such little care and review? Peanuts undergo far more examination by law, and they do not knock your socks off!

You could say, let them smoke themselves silly, what do I care? But once they use it with any regularity, they will develop "amotivational syndrome," become disabled, drive cars dangerously, end up in hospitals, and generally unemployed and unable to pay for medical care, living expenses, posing not only a danger to themselves, but to others as well. Even if they did have pain, and many do not, marijuana is not an effective pain medication, and is highly addicting. Most chronic users suffer from cannabis induced psychiatric and medical disorders, far worse than any claimed pain in most instances. As far as I can determine, all consequences result from marijuana addiction.

Believe or not, I didn't ever use much marijuana, only maybe one or two times. I didn't like the illegal aspect or getting "stoned," where I felt like I couldn't move, and everything slowed down to a crawl or less. It's just one addiction I managed to escape, but I had plenty of others. The prevalent view is marijuana is safe, painless, and not addicting. I can't think of anything much further from the truth. Marijuana addiction often is denied, minimized, and rationalized by political and unscientific views that marijuana is harmless, beneficial, not addicting, and has no serious adverse effects. However, looking at the evidence derived from clinical practice, scientific research and diagnostic criteria in the *Diagnostic and Statistical Manual*, marijuana is as highly addicting, incapacitating, harmful, and dangerous as any other drug of addiction.

In addition, marijuana is currently classified as a Schedule I drug that is legally defined as highly addicting without legitimate medical indications by the Controlled Substance Laws (CSL). CSL are based on scientific information, regulate production, distribution, and prohibit non-medical use of controlled substances. While recognizing its medical value and purposes for health and medical use, CSL balance a marijuana user's potential for abuse or addiction, liability, and safety.

The essential features of addictive use of marijuana, namely, preoccupation with acquiring, compulsive use, and relapse are readily apparent in objective assessments derived from review of the medical and scientific literature. Prevalence for use and dependence (addiction) to marijuana is frequent and widespread, and prevalence is indicative of preoccupation as in addictive use.

Despite the legal and medical evidence, I find many people claim marijuana is not addicting. What else could explain its widespread use, the most commonly used addicting drug in the world next to nicotine? Other than: addiction?

What should I be so surprised as cigarettes provide little or no benefit, yet are consumed addictively throughout the world. Add alcohol, and addiction looks like it makes the world go around without much benefit, other than maybe controlling population growth.

In the days working on an inpatient psychiatric unit, I observed a very consistent pattern over years, namely, positive urine drug screens for THC, (tetrahydocabinnol), which is the active ingredient in marijuana. I estimate that as many as a third of the psychiatric admissions were associated with regular marijuana use, often daily consumption. The chief complaints were often anxiety, depression, and suicidal behaviors. Sometimes paranoid beliefs and hallucinations. These complaints are often associated and caused by the chemical effects from marijuana but difficult for the user to comprehend due to its intoxicating effects.

When I tried to inform the patients that marijuana effects may be causing their psychiatric problems, they emphatically claimed that marijuana was helping with the anxiety and depression, even psychosis. It didn't seem to matter that they were admitted to a psychiatric hospital for suicidal behavior. They were totally resistant to the possibility that marijuana may be debilitating and killing them. Denial and poor insight and judgment are common in mentally ill patients, and particularly strong in marijuana users. Unless I was able to break through their denial, the prognosis is poor and disability while the risk of death continues.

Marijuana use historically begins at young age, though now later as well due to the availability of "medical marijuana." Psychiatric admissions for adolescents are commonly associated with marijuana use and it is assumed marijuana is part of the mental health problems. Unfortunately, it is viewed as a harmless drug, just incidental and not a problem, especially by physicians. Marijuana is also often found with other drug use, just adding to its dangerous effects.

An estimated 17% of past year marijuana users ages 12 and older used marijuana on 300 or more days within the past 12 months. This means that almost 5.4 million people used marijuana on a daily basis or almost daily basis over a 12-month period. An estimated 40.3% or 7.6 million current marijuana users age 12 and older used marijuana on 20 or more days in the past month. These criteria in aggregate and individually confirm a strong preoccupation with acquiring and using marijuana as in addictive use.

Epidemiological studies indicate that the past year prevalence of marijuana use was 9.5% in 2012 to 2013. A significant increase over the prevalence in 2001 to 2002, which was 4.1%. In addition, 7.22% of adolescent used marijuana in 2013-2014, which corresponds to approximately 1.8 million adolescent users. Risky behavior youth used marijuana in 2013 at a rate of 23.4%, more than three times the rate of the general population. In the past year, prevalence of DSM-4 marijuana use disorder was 1.5% in 2001 and 2002, and 2.9% in 2001 and 2003. In 2014, marijuana use disorder was 1.6%, which was consistent to the percentages for most years after 2005.

Certainly, medical marijuana has increased the prevalence of addiction and disability. Although medical marijuana is by state law decreed a medicine, there is no medical or legal basis for it qualifying as medicine. Review of the medical literature is void of studies to show its effectiveness. There are no controlled or even uncontrolled studies to show its effectiveness, and clinical experience and studies of addictive use confirm its ineffectiveness in any population or for any use.

The FDA has not investigated or approved marijuana for medical use. The FDA approves all medications for medical use and subjects a drug to rigorous, standardized testing before issuing approval to physician to prescribe. Therefore, physicians do not prescribe marijuana in medical practice. The Controlled Substance Laws classify marijuana as highly addicting and dangerous. As a Schedule I drug it has no legitimate medical purpose.

The medical marijuana laws were passed by the states, and are in conflict with federal law. Currently, the Federal Government only enforces federal marijuana laws if in violation of the state medical marijuana laws, assuming that the state laws are safe and effective, a rather arbitrary and unfounded assumption. The Federal Government totally ignores the addiction potential of marijuana and its adverse consequences. Any user is at risk for developing an addiction to marijuana, as many do. I struggle to understand why state laws allow marijuana use, as the states are supposedly responsible for the health and welfare of its citizens. Allowing almost indiscriminate use of marijuana to me is not in the interest of its citizens, even if the citizens want it.

However, the actual prevalence of marijuana addiction is likely much higher as over 50% of cannabis users appear to have impaired control over their use and symptoms of intoxication and withdrawal. Irritability, anxiety, craving, and disruptive sleep have been reported in 61-96% of cannabis users during intoxication and abstinence.

Public policy is based on public opinion, and is the basis for use and laws regarding marijuana. Contributing to the rise in prevalence in marijuana use and addiction is that Americans view drug abuse or drug problems as less important in recent years than in prior years. According to gallop polls between the early 1970s and the late 1970s, drug abuse was the most common and most important problem named by the public. Between 1979 and 1984, drug abuse did not appear at all in the gallop polls among the most often mentioned problems, indicating a relatively consistent low level of concern about the issue.

Not surprisingly, the support for the legalization of marijuana has conversely increased with decreasing public concern. In 1969, only 12% of the U.S. population supported the legalization of marijuana, according to a Gallop poll. By 2000, the support for marijuana legalization reached 30%. From 2000-2015, public support for the legalization of marijuana nearly doubled. In 2015, 58% of the population was in favor of marijuana legalization with 71% of young adults in support. The decrease in concern about marijuana use and the increase in support of marijuana legalization will undoubtedly result in increased marijuana addiction.

The compulsive use of marijuana is continued use, despite adverse consequences. These adverse consequences are a direct and indirect result of the marijuana addictive use, and not the cause of it. DSM-5 identifies and classifies the various states that collectively constitute adverse consequences from addictive use pertaining social, interpersonal, occupational, educational, legal, and medical adverse consequences. DSM-5 also contains diagnostic categories and criteria for cannabis intoxication, withdrawal and cannabis induced psychiatric states, anxiety, depression, and psychosis.

Cannabis is most commonly smoked via a variety of methods including pipes, water pipes, cigarettes (joints or reefers) or, more recently, in the paper of hallowed out cigars (blunts). Cannabis is also sometimes ingested orally, typically by mixing into food. More recently, devices have been developed in which cannabis is vaporized. Individuals with cannabis use disorder may use cannabis throughout the day over a period of months or years and thus, may spend many hours a day under the influence. Cannabis use affects work with repeated absences or increased risk working around dangerous situations. Arguments with spouses and other interpersonal relationship difficulties along with legal, medical, and mental health problems, can arise with cannabis use.

Importantly, whether or not cannabis is being used for "legitimate purposes," individuals who use cannabis are subject to and at high risk for developing a cannabis use disorder. Whether it is legal or illegal, use does not change the pharmacological properties of THC nor the addiction potential. In fact, legal use of medical marijuana contains high THC concentration and potency.

Compulsive use is demonstrated in the adverse consequences from accident and trauma due to marijuana use. The increasingly relaxed stance on marijuana only inflates the volume of accidents and subsequent trauma that result from marijuana. Montana Narcotics Chief, Mark Long stated, "DUI arrests involving marijuana have skyrocketed, as have traffic fatalities where marijuana was found in the system of one of the drivers." This statement has only been proven by the data. A study conducted by Students Against Destructive Decisions (SADD) found that driving under the influence of marijuana is currently a greater risk that drunk driving. In Washington State, cases where the driver tested positive for THC increased by 33% in the first six months of 2013. This is compared to a 7.9% decrease from 2011 to 2012. Additionally, Nevada's Traffic Bureau illustrates that from 2002 to 2012, 45% of drivers who were impaired by drugs had marijuana in their system.

Relapse, or an inability to abstain, is easily seen in the regular daily use of marijuana. Clinically, marijuana addiction is common among those who use daily, which indicates preoccupation/compulsive use. Marijuana can also be used more intermittently with adverse consequences, which would indicate a pattern of relapse as well. Of importance is the inability to abstain from marijuana, particularly in social, occupational, and legal situations, which increases the risk of dangerous outcomes and disability.

Specifically, for marijuana and disability, a study looked at the level of drug abuse among individuals enrolled in the Supplemental Security Income and Social Security Disability programs. Among these individuals, 23% had a lifetime dependency on marijuana, consistent with the various populations of federal aid recipients. This finding illustrates that almost one quarter of individuals receiving federal aid were using marijuana. This percentage will undeniably increase, as the marijuana is more easily accessible through legal means as with opioids.

The study also illustrated that the individuals that had the most difficulty obtaining work, were the group with the most psychiatric impairments. Marijuana use increases psychiatric impairments and is associated with psychiatric disorders at alarmingly high rates. Therefore, marijuana use leads to increased unemployment and disability resulting in extremely high costs not only to the individual, but also to the general public. As in the case of prescribed opiate use, marijuana is not a permanent and medically necessary disability under Social Security Disability and/or other forms of disability. Marijuana associated disability is reversible and improves or resolves with cessation of marijuana use.

Marijuana has been considered a gateway drug to other drugs, such as alcohol, heroin, or nicotine. There is a generalized vulnerability to addicting drugs including alcohol, and they are substituted and used interchangeably. The use of one addicting drug increases the probability of using another addicting drug. Marijuana use is highly correlated with alcohol, opioids (including heroin and prescription opioids), and cocaine use disorders. All of these drugs act through the mesolimbic reinforcement area in the brain and have a common pathway to addictive use. Predictably, use of one addicting drug, such as marijuana, leads to the use of additional addicting drugs as in a generalized vulnerability to drug addiction.

One such study illustrated the biological effects of THC on the brain. Adolescent rats, treated with THC, illustrated an upward shift of self-administered heroin throughout the study. Conversely, adolescent rats without the THC maintained the same pattern of heroin administration. This supported the hypothesis that adolescence marijuana use has an impact on hedonic processing that results in increased opiate intake, which could be the consequence of altering neurological pathways.

Additionally, another study examined the effects of marijuana use among twins. The study gathered information from sets of twin in which one twin used marijuana before age 17, while the other twin abstained from marijuana use before they were 17 years old. The study illustrated that the individuals that used marijuana prior to 17 years of age were 2.1 to 5.2 times higher than their co-twin to have other drug use, alcohol dependence, and drug abuse/dependence. This study clearly illustrates that early marijuana use increased a person's likelihood of using or abusing other drugs.

In order for marijuana to be a gateway drug, the use must be prior to the use of other drugs. In 2013, 70.3% of adult users of illicit drugs stated marijuana was their first illicit drug used. This fact alone is a strong indicator that marijuana is used as a gateway for use of other illicit drugs. Consistent with this statistic, studies of adolescent illicit drug use indicate that marijuana is used much more frequently by 12-17 year olds than other illicit drugs. In 2014, marijuana use by adolescents was at 7.4%, followed by nonmedical use of psychotherapeutics at 2.6%. Marijuana use at 7.4%, was higher than the percentage of other illicit drugs use by adolescents combined, which only totaled 4.0%.

Statistics also illustrate that marijuana use is also a gateway for tobacco use. As cited previously, adolescent marijuana use was 7.4% and adult marijuana use was 7.5%. Comparatively, cigarette use among adolescents was 5.6% and adult cigarette use was 21.3% in 2013. This indicates that while adolescents use marijuana in their youth, they add cigarettes as they grow older, which implicates marijuana as a gateway drug.

Overall, there is only evidence that prescription opioid medications are not effective when prescribed continuously for chronic pain. In fact, the evidence shows that opioids are less effective than non-opioid medications while being highly addicting and incapacitating. We have known for years that prescription opioid medications are highly addicting Schedule II drugs. We are experiencing an epidemic of death and disability from addiction to prescription opioid medications and their consequent cause of addiction to heroin and other drugs.

We are headed down the same path with marijuana, and have not yet learned that marijuana is similarly addicting. It is not effective in pain control and treatment of debilitating medical conditions, it is highly toxic and debilitating, and associated with promotion of other drug addictions such as heroin. Just as with opioids, marijuana is being touted as the answer to pain control and treatment of disabling conditions. That pain and suffering can be relieved by yet another addicting medication. If the facts mattered, and health was really the goal, we would not take that path to more marijuana.

Help, not just anybody
Help, you know I need someone, help

—"Help" The Beatles

21

IT GETS BETTER,
IT WORKS IF YOU WORK IT

"Do not lose courage in considering your own imperfections." —Saint Francis de Sales

Steps 10, 11, 12 are called maintenance steps. Meaning, I maintain my sobriety and abstinence through working these steps. I did the heaving lifting in steps 1-9, admitting my powerlessness in Step 1, restoring my sanity in Step 2, made a decision in Step 3, took a searching and moral inventory in Step 4, admitted to self, another, and God, the exact nature of my wrongs in Step 5, became entirely willing to have my character defects removed in Step 6, humbly asked Him to remove my shortcomings in Step 7, made of list of those I had harmed and became willing to make amends in Step 8, and made amends to them except when to do so would injure them or others in Step 9.

I have always questioned these steps but have also always worked them. They saved and continue to save my life. But as a scientist and medical doctor, I believe as firmly as I do in the steps, that addiction is a physical and mental disorder whose causes are located in the brain. Addiction, I always say, is a brain disease. So does the National Institute of Drug Abuse, the National Institute of Health, and the U.S. Government. Though addiction is brain in origin, we do not yet have effective medications to treat it beyond withdrawal. So I am left with believing that resentments, dishonesty, selfishness, anger, fear, impatience, and intolerance can lead to relapse to addictions. Though they do not create addictions. After over 30 years of recovery, I am not willing to abandon the use and practice of the 12 Steps. Certainly not for intellectual pride or doctor arrogance.

What do resentments, selfishness, anger, fear, impatience, and intolerance have to do with drinking and drugging? Damned if I know, but if they become too out of control, I am headed for trouble, big time. Not only will I run a collision course in dealing with others, and loss of serenity, I will risk relapse. Relapse is mysterious. Why would I want to give up all the mental and material gains from abstinence for a return to intoxication and hopelessness? I always say, AA will return your misery, don't worry. I have seen it happen over and over again, hard to escape. Relapse doesn't always happen right away, and in general the longer we are sober in AA, the longer relapse takes to occur. Relapse generally starts with a tapering of meeting attendance to an absence altogether, and gradually one day for no apparent reason, we take a drink. It may take a few years for this transitional slide to occur if one has been abstinent in AA for years. We lose our conditioning, and our negative emotions reemerge, and eventually we relapse.

In Step 10, I continue to keep aim, maintain self-analysis, and keep on the beam to stay abstinent from alcohol, drugs, debt, sex, though not perfectly. Step 10 says, "Continued to take personal inventory and when we were wrong promptly admitted it." A tall order in today's world. Not one that I meet ever completely. I remain driven by my instincts and compulsions, successes and defeats, focused and wandering. Most importantly, I continue to dream.

Without a dream, I lose hope, and without hope, I lose life. Without life, I lose thought, without thought, I lose existence. A famous French Philosopher proved his existence by saying "I think, therefore, I am." You see thinking is more than precious: it is priceless. You can't buy life.

Ever since that fateful day I made a "decision to live," I continue to reflect on life, liberty, and the pursuit of happiness. I could write a book on my mistakes, imperfections, and wrongs. Come to think of it, I did. But I am not very good at revealing my humanness. I have big doses of grandiosity and self-righteousness. One of my surest ways to avoid wrongs is to delay them. I try to wait before I act as long as I can. But it is also important to act.

That sequence is just the opposite of standard thinking, and traditional psychoanalytic thinking. Psychoanalysis instructs us to first change our feelings, then our thinking will change. Which then leads to a change in our behaviors or actions. Thus, introspection is the key. In 12-step recovery, while thinking is key, good thinking starts with right actions. A change in feelings is an end result, and not the start. Just the reverse of psychoanalysis. AA is an action program, beginning with the action of stopping drinking in Step 1, and continuing throughout the steps.

Recovery is action. I first act, stop drinking, then my thinking changes. Once my thinking changes, then my feelings change. Feelings are what drive me, both positive and negative. I act my way into right thinking, then the feelings follow, for better or worse. I am reminded about so many sayings that lifted and guided me during my early days of recovery. "Think, think, think," meaning try to remember how it was, what happened, and what it is like now. Denial is treading dangerous waters, and disguises the good, the bad, and the ugly from drugs and alcohol, so we think the opposite of what is actually true. Another is, "Nothing is so bad that a drink or drug won't make worse," meaning no matter how far down the scale we have gone or feel, a drink or a drug will not solve our problems, rather will make them worse. "Let go, let God," is one I use for cravings I may get though not often to use a drug or drink. Those urges I felt in early recovery were taken away by resorting to conscious asking for and turning my will over to God's help, and still central to my recovery. In fact, God is necessary. But remember that God is a short form for Good Orderly Direction, and is a Power I do not possess, which I can rely on for the strength I need to stay sober. And also to change, and keep changing, personally and professionally.

In Step 11, I maintain a conscious contact with that Power I lack. It says "Sought through prayer and meditation to improve our conscious contact with God as we understood Him, praying for knowledge of His will for us, and the power to carry that out." I do a daily prayer and reflection of sorts. I take time out in the morning before my day starts to read daily reflection books.

First I read the 24-hour book, which is about alcohol and spirituality. Then I read *The God Angle* which was written by an early founder and member of Alcoholics Anonymous. It starts out with a religious quote from the bible, and then applies it to alcoholism, AA, and recovery. Next is a book, *From the Heart*, which is about how spirituality can remove the isolation and bankruptcy from sex addiction. How I can fill my life with love and intimacy. The last book is *Food for Thought*, which is about being overweight and how I can control my eating and weight by filling my appetite with God and learn the difference between hunger and appetite. After all, addiction is out of control appetites and food is obviously linked to appetite.

Each book reminds me of my addictions, and asks me to commit to a daily reprieve from addictive drinking, drugs, sex, eating. A daily reprieve based on my spiritual condition. In a sense, I practice spiritual programs for each addiction daily, relying on 12 steps for each addiction. The concepts are the same for each addiction: powerlessness, sanity, decision to turn to God, take an inventory, admit to self, God and others, become willing to rid of character defects and humbly perpetuating my addictions, make amends from a list, and do it as promptly as I can. All while maintaining a conscious contact with a power greater than myself, and my spiritual awakening. One day at a time, I defend myself from the addictions, and grow in understanding and effectiveness in my adventure in my daily living. I solve my dilemma of powerlessness through spiritual practices.

I learned that my two worst enemies are yesterday and tomorrow. I cannot change the past, nor do I want to shut the door on it. But I cannot let the guilt haunt and destroy me, and lead me to drink or drug. I have steps to come to terms with the past, and actually use them as assets, as I try to help others while helping myself. I cannot mentally or spiritually live in the past without consequences, and practically speaking it does no good. Regrets, ruminations, and resentments don't take me far into the future, and hold me back from progress. Tomorrow is filled with apprehensions, fear, and projections paralyze me from moving ahead. I cannot make decisions based on reality that is not yet happening. Living in today is the best chance I have at abstinence, serenity, prosperity, abundance, fulfillment, love, and intimacy. Favorite sayings of mine are, "Just for today" and "One Day At a Time," for I can manage my challenges in a 24-hour period. Whereas, I cannot live in yesterday and tomorrow.

Getting down to the nitty gritty to pray for God's will for me and the power to carry it out is the really hard part. After I turn my will and my life over to the care of God, or Higher Power as I understand Him, now I have to pray for the knowledge of His will for me and the power to carry it out. All of this in the name of abstinence from my addictions. Why, you ask? Damned if I know, but it works. And this works for other things in my life. My personal life, family life, professional life. I learn to do this by practicing the steps.

While this step and the others sound and look religious and forbidding, they are not. They are a plan or blueprint for living, a practical guide and took kit to succeed. I am an ambitious type who wants to succeed, I don't want to become a monk and wear a sack cloth to learn God's will and do penance so that I am worthy. I want to live in the here and now, and find abundance and prosperity in my physical, mental and spiritual life.

If I am drinking and using addicting drugs, debting, overeating, and having indiscriminate sexual encounters, I am not likely to find peace, serenity, be able to work, earn and spend money sanely, be healthy and appear attractive, or find intimacy and love in a relationship. Addiction often becomes a physical, mental, and spiritual disease. Recovery motivates me improve all those conditions. I have chosen God's help for to do that. However, the steps are very practical, and provide actions that lead to changes in mind, body, and soul. I am not happy if I cannot change and become better. God or a higher power knows how I can change, I don't. I know God's will as I seek it, and ask for His power to carry it out. I learn by doing, and by doing I learn. I solve my dilemma of lack of power by seeking a Higher

Power.

In Step 12, I had a spiritual awakening. It says, *"Having had a spiritual awakening as a result of these steps, we tried to carry this message to alcoholics, and to practice these principles in all our affairs."* A spiritual awakening can take many forms. A sudden burst of lightening from God is unusual and dramatic spiritual awakening. A conversion based on hearing voices from God is another rare awakening mostly from the movies and novels. I always believed in God, but had a falling out with God in my freshman year of college when my early Judaic religious upbringing clashed with my later Catholic religious experiences. I could not reconcile a living Christ, and became deeply depressed, feeling abandoned.

I had used religion for years as a moral code for conscience and guidance in my everyday living. Religion has provided some kind of direction and filled a spiritual power most of my life. But I had reached an abyss, lost my being, and I became adrift in darkness in early college. I had become depressed, seriously. I had lost my power. That didn't change for some time, and when it did, I was hopelessly alcoholic. I had been overcome by emptiness and lack of spirit. I didn't totally lose my drive to succeed, just lost purpose.

When I made a decision to live and to recover in AA, I was told I needed a higher power, and that I could not do it on my own. I was also told that I would find that spiritual awakening as result of the first eleven steps. I had not come to terms with my conflict over Christian and Jewish religious practices and beliefs. For me, because recovery in AA and the 12 Steps was a practice over time, I gradually discovered a spiritual awakening with an occasional emotional boost. An uplift that one associates with a spiritual awakening. God was doing for me what I could not do for myself, e.g. not drink or drug. Another was a release from the God-awful guilt and condemnation from my past after making amends in the 9th Step. I could answer the phone without worrying if I had made a call in a blackout.

I soon realized in order to recover I had to acquire a "God-consciousness" in my own way. I acquired such a "God consciousness" by taking actions, learning as I did, and becoming aware of a power. My spiritual experiences were similar to what William James called the "educational variety," because they developed slowly over a period of time. I finally realized that I had undergone a profound alteration in my reaction to life. That such a change could hardly have occurred by myself alone. What took place in months I could not have accomplished by years studying philosophy, as I did.

In college, I had taken philosophy courses to try to find meaning, and God, to understand my existence, but came up short. I found more questions than answers, and no personal God or power to change me, or to help me stop drinking and drugging. I did not have the discipline to save my life. In recovery, I was able to find an inner resource, which I identified with my own conception of a Power greater than myself. To me, that Power greater than me is the essence of spiritual experience or God consciousness.

I can say with personal experience, that others can recover from alcoholism and drug addiction as I did and do. So long as I do not close my mind to all spiritual concepts, I can honestly face my problems in light of spiritual experiences. I can only be defeated by an attitude of intolerance or belligerent denial. Others can do the same. I can find and use this Power as I exercise the essentials of recovery, willingness, honesty, and open-mindedness. These are indispensable.

As a result of these steps, I try to carry this message to other addicts. In my early years of recovery, I worked on a personal level with alcoholics and drug addicts. As I gained more traction in my professional life, I withdrew from personal work with alcoholics. I found I could not completely separate my personal recovery from my patients' problems.

As a physician, I play a different role than I do as a recovering alcoholic. I also have different responsibilities and duties as a doctor than I do as personal advocate. Of no small measure, I have potentially tangible liabilities as a doctor that could intrude on personal obligations. Such as I could be sued as a doctor potentially, if I start to give medical advice even if on a personal level. It could be construed that I have a doctor-patient relationship with another alcoholic, even if I am interacting with personal intent.

Nonetheless, I have carried the message in my professional capacities, as physician and attorney. To what extent that aids or deters my personal recovery is a matter of thought and debate. I am still not sure. But I am sure I want to help those still suffering alcoholism and drug addiction as a physician and an attorney. I do that by working with them in clinical or treatment settings, which are psychiatric and medical. I also have written extensively in medical literature and done published research in addictions. Carrying the message is no easier professionally than personally, as I faced prejudice, bias, a lot of ignorance, as well as belligerence and denial (a lot). Missing are honesty, open mindedness and willingness.

I tried to change the plight of the alcoholic and addict as a physician through my medical care, publications, teaching, and as an attorney by suing doctors and hospitals.

I can't say I have been wildly successful, but I have made changes for the better in my own little world. Hospitals have altered their approach to medical care of addicts, providers do read my books and journal articles, and doctors and hospitals have been put on notice. Some doctors even changed their treatment practices and lost jobs as consequences of my lawsuits.

But the general public wants more addicting drugs, and gets them through the spurious medical route with increased prescribing and availability of addicting prescription opioids, narcotic medications. The so-called, "medical marijuana" is another path to intoxication and addiction that the public vigorously pursues. These drugs do not solve medical problems. Rather, they create them. Profit motives are always lurking as addictions generate more medical care for doctors and hospitals, and pharmaceutical companies can't make addicting drugs fast enough to match their greed.

The Industrial-Medical complex overall kills more than it saves lives when it comes to addicting drugs they push on to the public. The government caps it all off by making satisfaction a criterion in medical care, so that unsatisfied, demanding, and complaining addicts can cause a lot of problems in reimbursements. Remember, addictive drive and drug seeking is a self-fulfilling, pathological, and dangerous force that has little satisfying outcomes.

Furthermore, governments gain windfalls with sin taxes by taxing tobacco, alcohol, and now marijuana. What they don't realize is that destruction from medical and legal consequences result in a net loss in income, and good society. Supporting addicting drugs is not supporting the primary role of states to ensure the health, safety, and welfare of its citizens.

Addictions in the public are a lot like politics, where honesty is a liability, allegiance is more important than reality, and willingness only goes so far past self-interest. Addictions suffer from a blind, dumb, and lost public. One that wants more, not less addictions. Addictions cause over a million deaths per year, and billions in government costs to disability and entitlements. Not to mention the health care costs from addictions, and personal misery and suffering, much of it unnecessary. And regrettable and merciful deaths.

In order for me to stay sober, abstain from alcohol and drugs, not debt compulsively, and maintain satisfying sexual relationships, I must make recovery from these addictions my highest priorities. The rest of my life is contingent on and depends on, keeping these addictions in check, one day at a time. Having recovery first, makes all the rest possible. If I compulsively drink, drug, debt, or act out sexually, I jeopardize the rest of my priorities, support, satisfactions. According to my recovery, my family is my next priority. For me that means my daughters. My relationship with them is a life-long priority to support their health and welfare, intangibly and tangibly. I derive great joy from them. Next to my recovery, I have no greater obligation or satisfaction. And the more I demonstrate recovery to them, the better they do, I believe.

For whatever reasons, I did not share with them I was an alcoholic, drug addict until the older daughter was age 16. Given her genetic propensity and wild friends at the time, she was at risk for such an act of poor judgment. Almost immediately, I took her to an AA meeting where I gave an Open talk, and told my story. I also revealed my anonymity to my younger daughter at the same time. I told them about AA and my recovery, which to them fit my exhortations and cautions to them about alcohol and drugs. And I didn't drink or use drugs, so they probably suspected something. I am still not sure why I didn't tell them sooner except I had been sober for years when they were born, so they had no experiences with my addictions. I wanted to raise them in an addiction free environment, and accept me as a father. Their response when I told that was, "I am proud of you, Dad." *What more could I ask for?*

Later, my older daughter thanked me for my harping on her to avoid alcohol and its related consequences when she applied to medical school. She decided not to ride with her close friends to her High School prom because she knew they would drink alcohol, and they did and received misdemeanor charges for minor in possession. My daughter didn't drink and didn't have to report an MIP on her medical school application. She was thrilled and relieved. So was I. Thankfully she is now a resident in surgery, and understands some of the consequences of alcohol. She still drinks. I'll try to keep an eye on her. She has me as model, as she has used all her life.

My younger daughter shows signs of drug use though she seems to moderate it so far. I inform her as best as I can to help her avoid the consequences I faced from my drug use. She has some insight and understanding of the negative aspects but feels she can handle certain drugs, and gains something positive. She is otherwise responsible in other matters. And working on a career, though not in medicine, rather in a more creative avocation. Well suited to her talents, and ambitions. I am totally supportive of her goals and aspirations as I am with the older daughter. She is my daughter after all. She listens to me, though she doesn't like to admit it.

Although my career takes up a large amount of my

time, it is my third priority. Now that I am sober and am gifted in health, I can still work productively, with some choice of what I do. While my health is partly blessed by helpful genes, I take rigorous steps to keep and improve my health. I take no medications. I swim several times a week. I walk fairly often. I have arthritis, and have had 2 hip replacements. I have a tenuous back, but don't do all the exercises I need to do to strengthen it. My weight is over the recommended BMI, so I should lose some pounds for better mobility, and to avoid Diabetes Mellitus that runs in my family. But I struggle, as losing weight is as hard as sin. I watch my diet for calories and reduce how much I eat. I don't lose weight very fast, but I'm halfway to my goal. A characteristic that defines me is persistence, so I suspect I will make my desired, healthy, and comfortable weight someday before it is too late, I hope.

One of the co-founders of AA, Dr. Bob, always said, "Pass it on," and I try to do that in my personal and professional lives. It is a spiritual axiom that in order to keep my "Gift" of sobriety, I must give it away. Or I cannot keep it if I don't pass it on. I have learned and experienced in AA and other 12 Step programs, that "helping others" is my duty and joy. My work is devoted to finding ways to help others, while helping myself. I spend far more time helping others in my work. I am focused on helping all of my patients, clients, and colleagues, not just addictions. However, because I have special personal and professional knowledge, I provide viewpoints and perspectives that unfortunately are not seen commonly.

I analyze cases often where addiction to medications, marijuana, alcohol, and other drugs are overlooked. What happens is that patients with addictions and their effects go undiagnosed and their problems do not improve, such as medication induced depression. And insurance companies continue to pay unnecessary and costly claims, while employers pay for disability that is due to addicting medications; reversible and unnecessary. Medical care fraud is probably common as health care providers continue to prescribe disabling treatments that worsen care, particularly in cases that are litigated personal injury cases. Hospitals can count on return business from prior untreated admission due to patients' relapse to drugs and alcohol, with resumed crises, suicidality, depression, and anxiety. I have plenty of opportunity to carry the message, though it often ends up on deft ears.

I was doing a high number of independent medical evaluations on employers of a major health insurance company. They terminated my reviews because I identified too many "addiction" cases. You would think an insurance company would want to help people by providing proper diagnoses and treatments. Maybe the unions blocked our attempts to help these employees, or the insurance company didn't want to pay for addiction and detoxification services. That's dumb because the bill for untreated addictions continues to grow as long as the patients suffer from addiction induced illnesses. I keep chugging along and stay busy, doing what I can to help.

Now I know, "practicing these principles in all our affairs" is daunting and where I often fail. But it is not how many times you fail that counts, it is how many times you *try* that matters. Though I practice these 12 Steps in my daily life, I am by no means a saint by anyone's standards. I am still trying to stay one step ahead of my addictions though I do work Step 1 in AA perfectly by abstaining from alcohol and addicting drugs, and in DA by abstaining from compulsive debting. I am not as good at abstaining from compulsive eating and sex on the other hand.

However, I am an example for other alcoholics and drug addicts who want to recover, and for professionals who want to help their patients and clients who suffer from addictive illnesses. I write articles and books to help physicians and others who care for patients and clients with addictions. I give talks and teach medical students, residents, doctors, and anyone who wants to know and listen. I am considered an expert in a field where expertise is lacking, and not highly valued, unfortunately.

Yet I am grateful. I am blessed. I have turned a life-threatening disease into an asset. I found a power greater than myself: to help others. I don't always know where I am going, but I am not lost. I have good orderly direction. I can live more in the solution, less in the problem. I can help where sometimes no one else can. God is doing for me what I could not do for myself.

Keeping sober and abstinent are the most important things in my life. The most important decisions I ever made were my decisions to give up my addictions. I am convinced that my whole life depends on not taking that first drink, drug, or debt. Nothing is as important to me as my own sobriety and abstinence. Everything I have, my whole life, depend on those things. *Can I afford to forget these, even for one minute?*

I hope you don't mind that I put down in words
How wonderful life is while you're in the world

—"Your Song" Elton John

EPILOGUE:
12 PROMISES

If I am painstaking about this phase of my development, I was amazed even before I was halfway through. Einstein said, "Anyone who has never made a mistake has never tried anything new." My first realization is that I was managing to stay sober while attending AA when I could not before. An immediate benefit was that I could "show up" for work my personal life, most anything, whereas I often tried but was not successful and mostly frustrated at missed opportunities and failed efforts.

I could remember what I did, make commitments I could keep. I no longer felt useless and embarrassed. I could plan, wear clean clothes, regain self-respect and the respect of others. I no longer felt like the low life alcoholic I had envisioned as a child, the proverbial dirty old man in a trench coat who sat on a park bench and drank alcohol out of a brown paper bag. The worst possible being, who everyone looked down on.

I had felt God abandoned me. I was living in the abyss and failing. I had no idea I had failed God. I later found out He had not failed me. I had nowhere to go except up or out. And I had failed at death and at living. What a bind, cornered. Steps 1 and 2 were the beginning. I had to accept my powerlessness over alcohol and how unmanageable I had become. And come to believe that a power greater than myself could restore me to sanity. Insanity according to Albert Einstein, was doing the same thing over and over again and expecting different results.

We will know a new freedom and a new happiness. Einstein said, "That deep emotional conviction of the presence of a superior reasoning power, which is revealed in the incomprehensible universe, forms my idea of God." I was no longer chained to alcohol and drugs. I did not have a tether that kept me from exploring the world. In my drinking and drugging I kept holed up and withdrawn from everyone, not answering the phone or even looking at the mail. At least, I could participate in my work, life, liberty and the pursuit of happiness. I developed hope, enthusiasm, and excitement in the present and in the future. I could accept commitments and challenges, and actually accomplish them. I tried new and different projects, despair lifted, and I started to make progress without long delays or defeats. God was in charge ultimately, whether I liked it or not, and would determine my fate. I could accept or reject His will for me to find freedom or bondage.

Freedom from bondage was accepting myself and God's will for me. My bondage was addictions and self. I had no idea self was such a problem for me. I had become so self-absorbed and preoccupied, I thought very little of others. I projected my depressed mental state onto the world. I believed life was a shit sandwich, and I struggled for another bite, as every day I drank and drugged. Not what I had signed up for as an ambitious, young man.

We will not regret the past nor wish to shut the door on it. Einstein said, "The value of a man should be seen in what he gives and not in what he is able to receive." I never imagined that my drinking and drugging, with its sordid and dark past could become an asset. I realized that I had learned and experienced valuable lessons to offer to others, to help them with the same problems I had. Moreover, I accepted my life as an addict and stopped ruminating on its regrets.

Prior to my recovery, I was filled with regrets about myself personally and professionally. I didn't like being Jewish, I was raised by uneducated parents, did not live in an upscale house, did not belong to country clubs, did attend the best schools always, was not married, had no children, couldn't finish a residency, or keep a job. I certainly did not like being an alcoholic, and felt less than, inferior.

In recovery, I learned all these regrets were what made me a person as I was, and empowered me to help others with their regrets. I had joined the human race, and was just another imperfect soul seeking truth and purpose. I had lacked purpose in my drinking days, and now I had enthusiasm in my recovery. God forgave me as I forgave myself. I was the beginning and God, the end.

Einstein said, "Morality is of the highest importance —but for us, not for God." In my early recovery, I could not look people in the eye, even those I did not know nor had no experience with. I had accumulated shame over the years, that were condemning and overbearing, and incompatible with self. I recall having to look away, for no reasons at all. I had projected the shame from past on strangers in the present. I knew I had to do something about the guilt that hounded me. It nearly killed me more than once, and certainly condemned me to a life of futility and emptiness.

After I made amends in the 8th and 9th Steps, I cleared some of the wreckage of the past and the guilt it created. I could then look people in the eye, and did not have to look away because of my self-loathing. Hating oneself can become comfortable in a sick way, paralyzing and lethal. Suicide is always an option. Making amends however, releases hate, loathing, and is replaced by self-worth, meaning. So exciting, and freeing. A spiritual experience if I ever had one, uplifting and powerful. I grew to like a spiritual experience more than shame and pity.

We will comprehend the word serenity. We will know a new peace. Einstein said, "Peace cannot be kept by force; it can only be achieved by understanding." That "it is only to the individual that a soul is given." As I came to terms with who I was, I was not in constant conflict with myself first, and then with others. I don't know that I ever achieved serenity per say, the state of being calm, peaceful, and untroubled. But for sure, I am more serene than I was in the terror filled days of my addiction. I was always waiting for the other shoe to drop, for the guillotine to come down on me, for the gun to go off, and for end to arrive, sooner than later.

My peace in recovery definitely turned down the volume of my chaotic addiction days, I had a predictable life style where I could accurately connect consequences to my actions, rather than random adversity from intoxication and blackouts. I now had a power greater than myself to rely on and I did not have to do it myself, alone. Instead of being at war with world, I now wanted to work with the whole. However, I was grandiose enough to want to change the world. And still do. I realized, though, I would make more progress if I changed me. Not as much fun, but more challenging and lasting. The 12 Steps were my means to change me.

No matter how far down the scale I have gone, we will see how my experience will benefit others. Einstein said the only source of knowledge is experience. I now had purpose and meaning, as I could help others similarly situated. That I was an alcoholic and even drug addict, choosing to help those who were confused and downtrodden, and addicted as I had been. I could relate to anyone who had my addiction problems, whether high or low. I could identify with powerlessness and unmanageability from the alcohol and drug addictions, and hopelessness. I had the same feelings from my addictions that others had, and I could identify with them. I learned early on that I should look for likeness, and not differences. Identification not comparison, is how we understand our addictions and gain strength to admit and accept our problems. We identify with others to recover, and see where our experiences will benefit others and ourselves. Even after many years I can benefit from hearing about the same experiences, and how others overcome and recover.

Personal responsibility is the cornerstone of recovery. I benefit so much from hearing how others accept responsibility for their addictive diseases in order to change. I am reminded that I cannot recover alone, I need help from others, and power of identification. Imagine I improve my self-worth from working with addicts and alcoholics, personally and professionally. I didn't plan on any of that when I started dreaming about my future. My ambitions did not include what many people consider low life. Nor did I ever think working with unfortunates would exalt my spiritually. Never did I think I could want to help others, I always am looking to help myself. But I do that with my Higher Power when I remember.

That feeling of uselessness and self-pity will disappear. Einstein said, "No problem can be solved from the same level of consciousness that created it." Sober, I started showing up to my clinical rotations in Neurology, instead of calling in sick or just not showing up at all. I began feeling self-respect already. Being a physician was certainly a boost, now that I could fulfill that role. I never respected myself drunk and hung over, or drugged and depressed. Addiction has a way of hollowing out self, leaving self on empty, meaningless, purposeless, wandering longingly. In Step 3, making a decision to turn my life and my will over to the care of God as I understood Him was the turning point that got me going to fill the abyss.

We will lose interest in selfish things and gain interest in our fellows. Einstein said, "Strive not to be a success, but rather to be of value." Self was my predominant mode in addiction life. I had little regard or concern about others. My motto was to help myself, first and last. My recovery teaches me that I will forget myself if I gain interest in others. Saint Francis Assissi's Prayer personifies how this works, "Lord, make me an instrument of thy peace. Where there is hatred, let me sow love; Where there is injury, pardon; Where there is doubt, faith; Where there is despair, hope; Where there is darkness, light; here there is sadness, joy."

Without question these are tall goals, unreachable by myself and most, and hard to do by any human measure. Do I even try? Maybe. I do it best when working personally or professionally with other alcoholics and drug addicts. I love, not hate addicts, with faith in power to stop the addiction cycle and hope instead of despair from addictive use. The 12 Step recovery provides practical suggestions to find a way of life and joy in personal change and growth, in order to live without that God-awful compulsion to use drugs and alcohol.

Self-seeking with slip away. Our whole attitude and outlook on life will change. Einstein said, "Without deep reflection one knows from daily life that one exists for other people. Coincidence is God's way of remaining anonymous." While recovery is "me first" and is a selfish program,

I am supposed to and do live according to spiritual principles, though not on a saintly level. Recovering people often claim there are no coincidences in daily living, just God's will acting for us and in us. As you know, I no longer want to kill myself. I want to live, and live abundantly. I show up and perform. Where I could not plan for the future because I could not predict my behaviors, I can now count on being clear headed, and live out plans as I make them.

Fear of people and economic insecurity will leave us. Einstein said, "To keep your balance, you must keep moving." I can't say that fear of people has completely left me, but I don't have the guilt and resentments that alienate me from people. I have a great deal more confidence that I will show up, accept challenges, and be responsible. "I am responsible" is a mainstay of my personal recovery in AA.

I still can't shake completely my fear of economic insecurity, but my recovery in Debtors Anonymous gives me suggestions, tools and steps, along with participation with other debtors in recovery. I certainly have more confidence in my financial decisions, and do not accumulate unsecured debt, and really not much secured debt because I still have to pay it back. I continue to increase my overall net worth, I continue to advance my career goals and increase my earnings. I save money and make much smarter investment decisions, and certainly understand them better. I spend money a whole lot better, and my earnings tripled and quadrupled in DA. I am not a billionaire yet, but have not given up hope. I live prosperously with much good fortune, not always monetarily.

We will intuitively know how to handle situations which used to baffle us. Einstein said, "Only two things are infinite, the universe and human stupidity, and I'm not sure about the former." My grandiosity may interfere with my intuition at times, and I mix up my dreams with reality, but I have tools to figure out solutions. I live much more in the solutions than in the problems. My judgment gets mixed up with my self-righteousness, and I expect the world to do the right thing. When it often ignores justice. Just how the medical profession can almost totally ignore addictions, marginalizes it, and can rationalize pain and suffering and death from addictions, continues to baffle me. The medical professionals and general public's stupidity in regards to drug and alcohol addiction may very well exceed the universe in magnitude.

We will suddenly realize God is doing for me what I could not do for myself. Einstein said, "We cannot solve our problems with the same thinking we used when we created them." This is where I step aside and ask for God's will to guide me in life. I recall when I first felt God was doing for me what I could not do for myself, I had completed a trip of amends to Johns Hopkins Hospital. There I faced my near fatal overdose, met with my faculty, and told them about my recovery in AA. I had been sober for two years. The Department of Psychiatry accepted me back to complete my residency in Psychiatry. That was a personal achievement. My Chair accepted me back with open arms, and welcomed me back to my friends. I can't tell you how much that meant to me. And this came from a man who did not consider addiction a disease, but was certainly accepting of addicts. Man's Best Hospital that saved my life, and gave me back my soul.

Are these extravagant promises? I think not. They are being fulfilled within me, sometimes quickly, sometimes slowly. They will always materialize if I work for them. For me, I have worked the programs of Alcoholics Anonymous, and more recently Debtors Anonymous, and have realized sooner or later my goals and aspirations. I am truly blessed, by my Aristotle's Unmoved Mover. The 12 Step programs fit the Unmoved Mover because I must seek and work the steps, and take actions daily to achieve outcomes. I cannot wait for God to come to me, I go to God. Ultimately, I find the power I lack, to abstain and to live within my old skin, and reconcile my conscience with the world, and mostly importantly myself.

All you need is love, love
Love is all you need

—"All You Need Is Love" The Beatles

REFERENCES

To find the information quoted by the author throughout this book on Alcoholics Anonymous, including *12 Steps, 12 Traditions* and *The Big Book of Alcoholics Anonymous*, please go to: http://www.aa.org.

The Diagnostic and Statistical Manual of Medical Disorders (DSM-5) can be found in bookstores or on several websites, including http://www.psychiatry.org.

Answers in the Heart: Daily Meditations for Men and Women recovering from Sex Addiction, author anonymous, can be found on Amazon.com.

The God Angle by Robbie R., 2017. can be found on Amazon.com

Food for Thought: Daily Meditations for Overeaters by Elisabeth L., can be found on Amazon.com

CITATIONS

Astrachan, B., Hoffman, N., Miller, N., Ninonvuevo, F., "Lifetime Diagnosis of Major Depression as a Multivariate Predictor of Treatment Outcomes for Inpatients with Substance Use Disorders from Abstinence-Based Programs." Annals of Clinical Psychiatry. 1997:9 (3): 127-137.

Blanco, C., Hasin, D., Wall, M., et al. "Cannabis Use and Risk of Psychiatric Disorders." JAMA. 2016.

Brown, T., Hartman, R., Milavetz, G., et al. "Cannabis effects on driving lateral control with and without alcohol." Drug and Alcohol Dependence. 2015: 154:25-37

"In U.S., 58% Black Legal Marijuana Use." http://www.gallup.com/poll/186260.

"Marijuana Use and Perceptions of Risk and Harm from Marijuana Use: 2013 and 2014." https://www.samhsa.gov/data/sites.

National Institute on Drug Abuse. "Drug Facts: Nationwide Trend." https://www.drugabuse.gov/publications/drugfacts/nationwide trend

ABOUT
THE AUTHOR

Bohunk is a doctor and attorney with board certifications and clinical practice in Addiction and Forensic Psychiatry, as well as Neurology. He is a respected authority and prolific author, as well as a highly valued expert witness and popular guest lecturer. *Bohunk*'s commitment to educating the public and helping the addicted has become his life's work. In sharing this story he retains his anonymity, in respect to Tradition 11 of Alcoholics Anonymous.

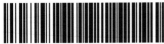

Made in the USA
Middletown, DE
09 June 2019